TOMORROW'S WORLD **MEDICINE**

DO NOT REMOVE
CARDS FROM POCKET

ALLEN COUNTY PUBLIC LIBRARY

FORT WAYNE, INDIANA 46802

You may return this book to any agency, branch,
or bookmobile of the Allen County Public Library.

DEMCO

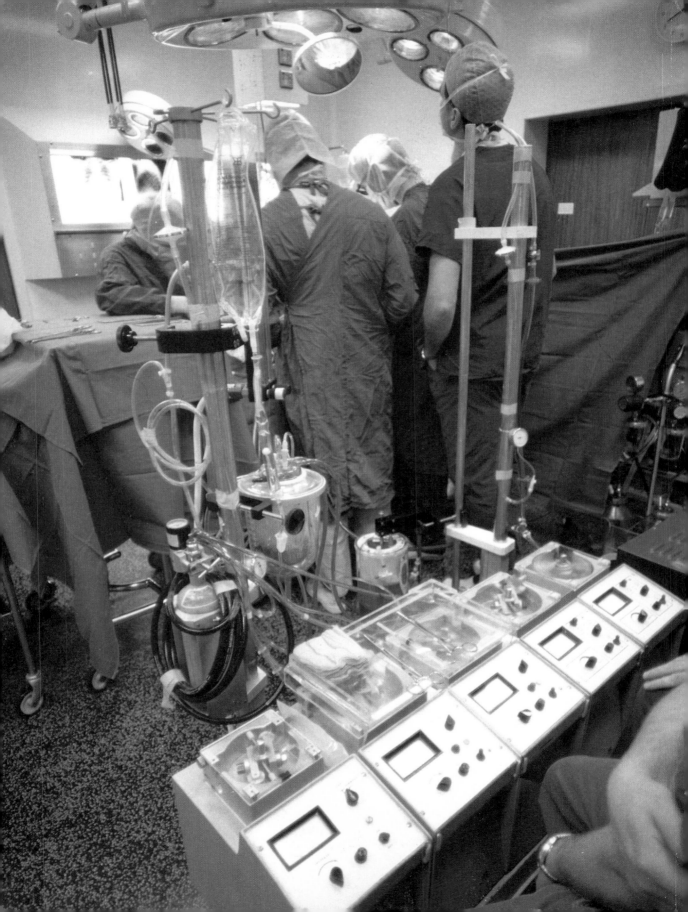

TOMORROW'S WORLD
Medicine

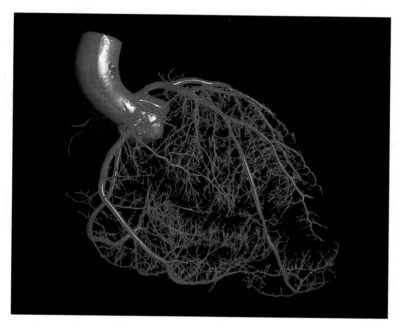

Fiona Holmes

British Broadcasting Corporation

With grateful thanks to the many doctors and medical scientists, too numerous to name, who helped me with advice and illustrations

Tomorrow's World was first broadcast on BBC 1 in 1965 and has been screened every year since then.

Published by the British Broadcasting Corporation
35 Marylebone High Street, London W1M 4AA

This book was designed and produced by
The Oregon Press Limited, Faraday House,
8 Charing Cross Road, London WC2H 0HG

ISBN 0 563 20344 7 hardback
ISBN 0 563 20346 3 paperback

First published 1985
© The British Broadcasting Corporaton 1985

Design: Martin Bristow
Picture research: Marion Pullen
Reader: Raymond Kaye

Filmset by SX Composing Ltd, Rayleigh, England
Printed and bound by Printer Industria Grafica SA,
Barcelona   D.L.B. 23766-1985

FRONTISPIECE The heart and lungs were among the earliest human organs to be temporally replaced by machines (*see Chapter Seven*)

TITLE PAGE The blood vessels of the heart (*see Chapter Seven*)

Contents

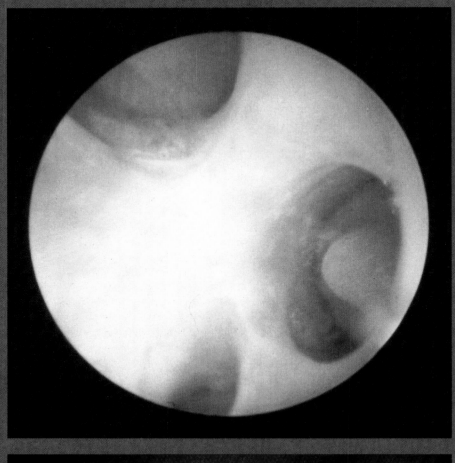
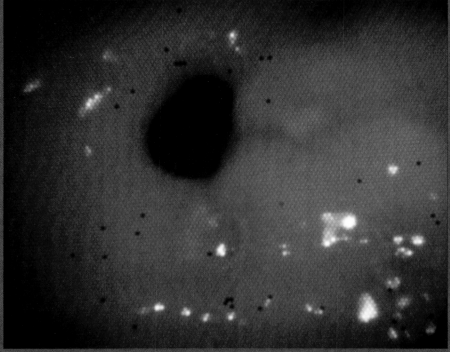

CHAPTER ONE
Know Your Enemy

Diagnosis

If you look at a register of deaths in London a century ago, you will find that there was one common cause of death that is very uncommon now. Many people died as a result of an 'act of God'. It seems unlikely that this change is due to a reduction in divine intervention, which means it must be due to improved diagnosis. Diagnosis is important not as an end in itself, but mainly because it may suggest a cause and a form of treatment: preferably leading to a cure. There are still times when the complaint is a symptom and the underlying cause is obscure. Then if it is not too serious, and particularly if it goes away of its own accord, medical honour is satisfied with a diagnosis like neuralgia (pain originating in a nerve), arthritis (inflammation of a joint), pityriasis rosea (pink spots). A classical education is a wonderful thing.

Other more serious problems also defy explanation, and then they are not only a cause of deep distress to the sufferers, they are also a severe thorn in the flesh of doctors. One such problem is Cot Death, or Sudden Infant Death Syndrome, when an apparently healthy infant dies suddenly without warning. There have been any number of suggestions about the cause, but so far pathologists have failed to show any consistent abnormalities that seem serious enough to cause the disaster. Epidemiologists have hunted for some recurring factor in the background of the babies, but although it happens more often among infants who are being brought up in difficult conditions, it certainly is not always so. Viruses have been blamed, chemical faults in the babies' lung development, accidental suffocation – it is still a mystery. Without an explanation doctors are powerless to prevent it, and one particularly tragic British mother lost four babies in the same mysterious way.

Fortunately the number of totally unexplained diseases is shrinking. Most disease can now be diagnosed to a degree that is more than just a description of the obvious symptoms, thanks to the invention of a range of tools, beginning with the stethoscope, which allows doctors to listen to the principal components of the heartbeat and noises in the lungs. It is still the doctor's badge of office, although now there are much more informative ways not only of listening to the body, but also of looking into it.

Inside information

It is a long time since asking you to say 'ninety-nine' gave a doctor the best view he was likely to get into your throat. Now any body cavity that has a natural entry or exit – and a fair number that have not – are accessible for inspection.

It is the development of the endoscope that has made this possible. The endoscope is a telescope for looking inside the body; there is a whole family of them, each with a different name derived from the part of the body it is designed to investigate. So there is a gastroscope for the stomach, a bronchoscope for the bronchi, or lungs, a nephroscope for

ABOVE A rigid endoscope looks into a kidney, showing the branching tubes where urine is collected.
BELOW A flexible endoscope shows the pylorus (the opening between the stomach and duodenum). There are two small ulcers, one to the right of the opening and one below it. The tiny black dots show where individual fibres in the bundle of 10,000 have been damaged

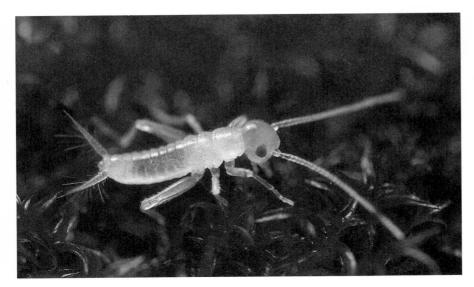

The cold light developed for endoscopes has other uses, such as in filming tiny delicate creatures that might die in too hot a light. This baby cricket is less than 2 mm long

the kidney, and a laparoscope from the medical jargon word for the abdomen. Some of these 'scopes are rigid tubes, some are flexible, depending on how easy it is to gain access to the affected part, and also depending on how important it is that the quality of the picture should be very good: because optically, the rigid 'scopes are certainly much better.

The ancestors of the modern endoscope were metal tubes with a small light bulb at the business end to illuminate the area to be examined, and a series of lenses spaced out along the tube to bring the picture back to the eyepiece. It was not a particularly good picture, since the light levels were necessarily low. The size of the bulb was very limited because it went inside the patient, and too hot a light would risk burning any delicate tissues it might touch. The invention of fibre optics transformed the endoscope, both by improving the existing rigid instruments, and by making it possible to produce flexible 'scopes.

In all endoscopes optical fibres are now used to carry the light, and because there is no longer any need for the source to go inside the patient much higher levels of light can be used. Also an ingenious mirror system is used to focus the light from the source into the optical fibres, and in the process to keep the light cool. This is what is known as a 'cold mirror'. The surface is made up of a number of thin films which are so arranged that the mirror reflects almost all of the light in the visible spectrum, but only a small part (about 20 per cent) of the infra-red. The light that reaches the tip of the 'scope inside the patient is thus much cooler than the source. The bundle of fibres that carries the light takes up about 20 per cent of the diameter of the telescope. The rest of the space is available for other things, like the lens system that carries the picture, and for one or more channels for instruments.

The rigid endoscope is a metal tube containing a series of lenses. Obviously it is limited in its use to parts that are accessible in a straight line from outside, but it does give a much better view than the flexible endoscope, particularly since the introduction of rod lenses.

If you think about it, it is obviously very difficult to fit the lenses accurately. You have a tube something like 300 mm (12 in) long, with lenses fitted at intervals all the way along it, and the diameter of the lens channel is something like 3 mm (0.08 in). Unless each lens is lined up with perfect accuracy the optics will be a disaster. The only way this can be done satisfactorily is by fixing the lenses first into a flexible inner tube and then threading that through the outer metal sheath. Since the total diameter of the endoscope has to be kept as small as possible, this loss of space is a serious disadvantage. With this type of arrangement the light getting back is still too dim to allow good photographs to be taken, and these are essential for accurate records as well as research work.

Rod lenses

The solution to the problem was found by Harry Hopkins, Professor of Optics at Reading University in Berkshire. What he suggested was that the manufacturers of endoscopes should reverse their existing procedure. Instead of a tube full of air with occasional glass lenses, they should produce a tube full of glass with occasional air 'lenses'. This had two advantages. For a start, it would be as difficult to get the alignment of these lenses wrong as it had previously been to get it right; so there would be no need for the inner tube, and the full space could be devoted to the lens. But a greater advantage would come from the fact that glass has a higher refractive index than air, and since most of the time the light would now be travelling through glass, much more would be transmitted. With extra refinements like special coatings on the surfaces, the rod lens endoscope has now been shown to let through 80 times as much light as the ones made by the old system.

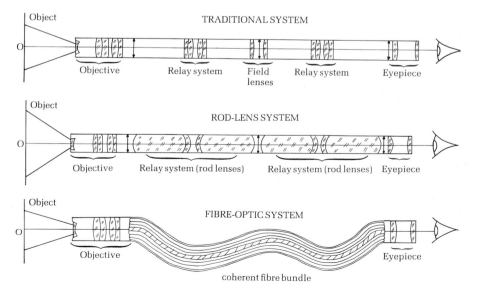

How the picture is transferred to the eye in three different types of endoscope. A bundle of fibres carrying the light travels alongside the lens channels

The flexible approach

Many parts of the body, like most of the lungs and the stomach, are not accessible to the rigid endoscope. Hence the need for flexible 'scopes, where the only lenses are at the two ends of the instrument; in between there is a bundle of optical fibres, each one carrying a tiny portion of the picture. Unlike the bundle of fibres that carries the light, this of course has to be very carefully arranged in what is known as a coherent bundle. Each fibre must emerge from the bundle in precisely the same relation to all the others as it went in, otherwise the picture will make total nonsense. In any case the picture always emerges as a matrix of separate dots, and focus is not usually as good as the lens system, so for observing minute detail the rigid type is better. However, the flexible endoscope makes up for this by its ability to reach the parts other 'scopes cannot reach, since it will work perfectly satisfactorily up to 2 m (78 in) long.

In addition to the light bundle and the part of the tube occupied by lenses or optical fibres, space is left for at least one more channel, sometimes two. These are the instrument channels, and a full kit of remotely controlled tools has been developed to operate through endo-scopes. A great many surgical procedures are now done this way (see Chapter Five), but there are also tools that are used to help in diagnosis. One channel may be needed simply to pour down water or other fluid to wash the lens or the area being examined, perhaps because blood is spoiling the view. Or in the reverse direction the same channel may be used to suck up excess fluid, or to take a sample of mucus or surface cells – from the lungs for instance. Should a larger sample of tissue be needed for examination in the laboratory, there are small pincers and snares that can nip off a tiny piece. Study of tissues samples is often the only way of telling what a tumour is, and whether there is a suitable treatment, and to obtain such a sample in the past would have meant an exploratory operation.

Examination of tissue samples is just one small part of the massive contribution of the scientist in the hospital laboratory to the diagnosis of disease. Until the end of the nineteenth century doctors did all their own laboratory work. It was mainly done on urine because until the hypodermic syringe became generally available in the 1920s, taking a blood sample involved cutting down to a vein and cupping (covering the incision with a warmed glass cup which would draw out the blood as it cooled). For most doctors urine analysis meant observing its appearance, smell and taste. This last was to check for sweetness; sugar in the urine was known to be a bad sign as long as 1500 years ago, when it was noticed that ants were attracted to the urine of some sick people. Although urine is still very informative, the blood is much more so.

The message in the blood

There are three major groups of blood particles: red cells, white cells, and platelets. The platelets are small particles with no nucleus and their

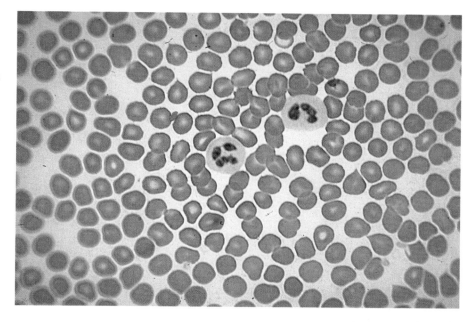

Human red blood cells, with two of the larger white cells in the centre of the picture

function is to stick together and patch up wounds. Red cells are the oxygen carriers; when mature they also contain no nucleus, but are packed full of haemoglobin, a large molecule that carries oxygen around the body. The last group, the white cells, is a collection of five different types of cell associated with the immune system. The proportion of the various cells in the blood is fairly constant in healthy people, but can change considerably in illness, so counting them can tell doctors a great deal. Anaemia, a disease in which the number of red cells falls dramatically, was one of the first non-infectious diseases to be scientifically treated – with supplements of vitamin B_{12}. The size of individual cells can be significant as well, because in different types of anaemia the blood cells can be larger or smaller than normal.

Thirty years ago if you had walked into a haematology laboratory you would have seen a row of people looking down microscopes, and the only noise would have been from counters in their hands, clicking away as they counted blood cells. Now this work can be done by machine. The blood is diluted and passed through tiny apertures that allow only one cell to pass at a time. As each cell passes through the aperture it causes a measurable change in resistance, and since this change is different for different volumes of cell it gives a measure of number and of size. The white cells present a bit more of a problem, because their numbers are so small that they are totally swamped by the red cells. To get over that the machine adds to the sample a chemical that will break down the outer walls of cells, but will not damage the nucleus. The white cells are the only blood cells with a nucleus, so the red cells and platelets are reduced to mush and then all the machine has to do is count nuclei. And since the nucleus of each of the main types of white cell is of a different size, they are sorted and counted in one process.

The remaining part of the blood, the liquid, is called plasma. This is 92 per cent water and the remaining 8 per cent is a mixture of nutrients, waste products, essential components like calcium, sodium, potassium, fats, enzymes, hormones, etc. Just as a shortage or excess of blood cells can result in disease, so can an abnormal amount of one of the ingredients of plasma. The plasma has therefore to be analysed, using a variety of chemical techniques. One is spectroscopy; in this the plasma is mixed with a range of chemical reagents that produce changes in colour which are measured. Electrophoresis is used to separate out the different classes of proteins. This is a technique where a tiny quantity of material is put at one end of a strip of paper or cellulose acetate and a current is passed through it. The proteins will move across at different speeds, according to their electric charge.

In practice most of these tests, just like the blood cell ones, have been highly mechanized, although critical judgments are still usually in human hands. But mechanization, and recent developments in micro-miniaturization, mean that some of the tests have found their way back out of the laboratory into the hands of doctors again. It is important that tests like those for blood gases and blood acidity (oxygen, CO_2 and hydrogen ions can be measured in arterial blood) are done as quickly as possible after the sample is taken, so with the help of automated equipment they are now done on the hospital ward, or at least in intensive care units.

Radiography: X-rays

The physicists entered medicine in a big way in 1895 when the German physicist Wilhelm Konrad von Röntgen showed the X-ray of his hand to the Physical Medical Society of Würzburg. For the first time the human body had become transparent. The early X-rays were only able to show large differences in density, so solid objects like bones were outlined. Modern results would look miraculous to the pioneers, but even so there are limitations to the information X-ray pictures can provide, and other systems are now being developed to make the body transparent in different ways. Nevertheless X-rays were the first, and they are still extremely useful.

X-rays can only distinguish between different densities of the tissue in the body they pass through. The X-ray tube, normally a tungsten source bombarded by a stream of electrons, emits a beam of X-rays which are directed on to the body, or part of the body, being investigated. Behind the body is a fluorescent screen, and in contact with the screen a photographic plate. Every time an X-ray hits the screen it fluoresces, and the light produces a darkened area on the photographic plate. The amount of radiation that gets to the fluorescent screen depends on how much is absorbed or scattered by the material in the body it passes through. Bone is a very dense material – the calcium it contains is an efficient absorber of X-rays – so very little passes and the bone appears as a sharp silhouette. Air, on the other hand, absorbs very little, so lungs or other air-filled spaces, like sinuses in the head or pockets of

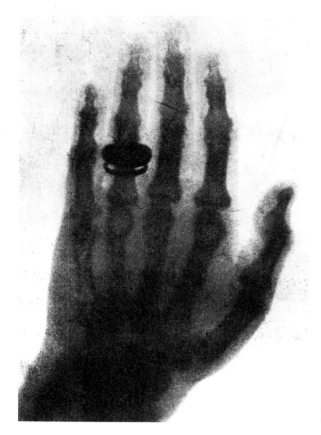

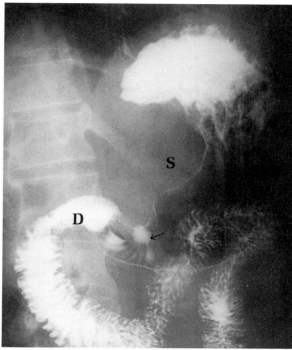

ABOVE LEFT The world's first x-ray picture, Röntgen's photograph of his own hand
ABOVE RIGHT X-ray following a barium meal. Most of the barium (showing white) has been expelled from the stomach – S – into the duodenum – D. A small amount has remained to reveal the crater of the ulcer (arrowed)

air in the gut, will show as less dense than the surrounding tissue.

One fact that limits the usefulness of a normal X-ray picture is that it is, of course, a two-dimensional portrait of a three-dimensional object. The rays are not focused at a chosen depth into the body, so anything in front of or behind a bone will be hidden in the bone's shadow. And because the number of photons arriving at the screen will be affected by the number absorbed on the complete journey through the body, small differences in tissue density will not be detectable.

The first half century

For the first 50 years or so following their discovery, X-rays in medicine were mainly used to look for broken bones, and to detect signs of lung disease. During both the First and Second World Wars, mobile X-ray units were used in field hospitals to look for lodged bullets and pieces of shrapnel – which showed up even more clearly than bones. In peace-time the mobile units travelled the country scanning the population for early signs of tuberculosis, which was still widespread.

Although they were good at producing pictures of lungs and bones, X-rays gave very little information about anything else, until it occurred to radiologists that it would be possible to make other parts of the body just as visible by filling them with a substance that would be opaque to the rays in the same way as bones were. The higher the atomic number of an element, the more X-rays it will absorb, so barium, in the harmless

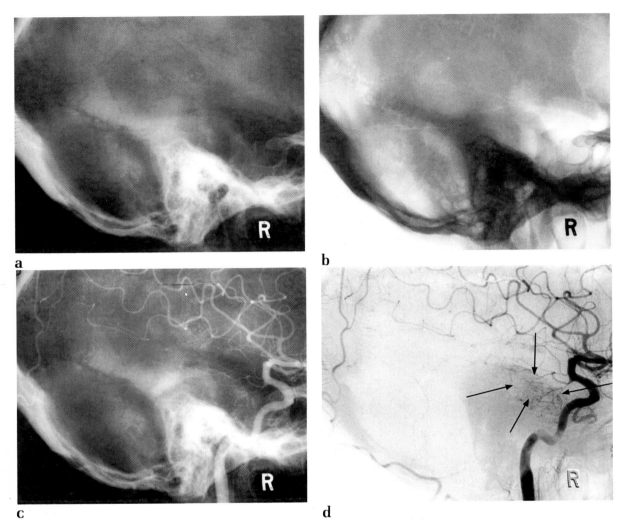

a

b

c

d

compound barium sulphate, was swallowed to fill the upper part of the digestive tract, or given as an enema to outline the lower. With the tract full of barium any ulcer, tumour or other obstruction would show as a distortion of the outline. In the same way, individual blood vessels can be clearly outlined by injecting iodine, another radio-opaque element. This technique has been refined to such a degree that a single vessel, or the branching vessels feeding a tumour, can be isolated and outlined. Since iodine is carried quickly through the vessels, by taking a series of still pictures or by using cine film, the flow of the blood through the vessels can be shown exactly as it happens. By attaching the iodine to various molecules that are known to be absorbed in specific parts of the body, the same technique can be used to produce good pictures of the kidneys, bladder, gallbladder, lymph nodes, etc.

There are two main difficulties with these procedures. One is that the bones and other structures tend to get in the way of clear interpretation of the picture. The second is that the contrast medium, the fluid containing the iodine, causes discomfort, a burning sensation, and in a very few people a more severe reaction.

(a) An x-ray of part of the skull. Picture taken before injection of contrast medium.
(b) Negative of above.
(c) Contrast medium now outlines blood vessels, but picture is confused by bone.
(d) After subtraction of (a), the picture clearly shows blood vessels feeding a tumour (arrowed)

The usual way of solving the first problem is by taking one master shot before injection of the contrast. Then, after the contrast has been injected, a series of further pictures is taken. When they have all been processed a negative is made of the first, master, shot, and this is used as a mask to 'subtract' all the solid structures that are there all the time, and are therefore of no interest. The resulting plates should show only the contrast-outlined blood vessels. The only problem with this system is that it is laborious, and the radiologist cannot be certain that the pictures are satisfactory until the whole double development procedure has been gone through: the poor patient may therefore have to remain on the table all the time this is being done.

Digital vascular imaging

DVI promises not only to make the 'subtraction' procedure immediate, but also to reduce the difficulties with the contrast medium. Instead of the fluorescent screen, the X-rays are collected by an electronic image intensifier, and the pictures are shown on a television screen rather than film.

The camera first of all takes a shot to use as the mask. This is stored in the machine's computer, and will be automatically subtracted from any pictures shown on the monitor thereafter. So when the contrast is injected, subtracted pictures are produced at once and are stored on disc. Sometimes the patient will move slightly during the time when the contrast is being injected, which means that the subtraction is not quite as good as it might be. With the electronic system this is no problem, because it is possible simply to select a later frame, after the

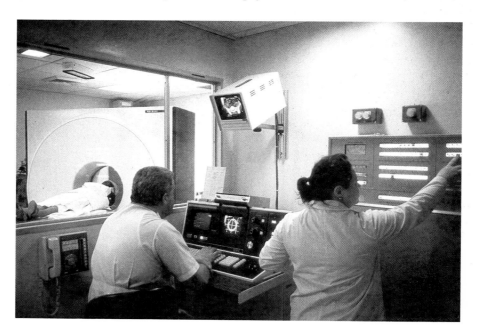

A brain scanner in use. The principle of producing pictures from scanners of this type was developed by EMI Ltd in 1971

move, and tell the computer to re-process the subsequent frames using the later shot as mask, instead of the earlier one. Unlike the film technique this takes a matter of seconds. But from the patient's point of view the biggest advantage of the electronic system is that it is much more sensitive than film, so much weaker contrast solution can be used. To produce a film picture of the arteries leading to the kidney, for instance, it would be necessary to thread a tube through the blood vessels to a precise spot alongside the kidney before injecting. Now it is possible to inject the contrast through a needle into the arm, much less unnerving for the patient; and even then the solution can be weaker than is needed for the older system.

For all its refinement, the DVI image is still a two-dimensional picture of a three-dimensional object. CAT scanning gives a two-dimensional picture of a two-dimensional slice.

Computed axial tomography
In the CAT scanner the patient lies with his body, or head, through the middle of a hoop. An X-ray source on one side of the hoop produces a narrow beam which passes through the body and is picked up by detectors on the far side. The source travels around the circle, and either there is a full round of detectors opposite or the same row of detectors travels around in synchronization with the source. In either case the information from the detectors is fed to a computer, which builds up a picture of the slice by comparing the signal received in each of the positions (sometimes as many as a thousand) and calculating what the contribution of each point on the slice must be to produce that particular overall pattern of signals.

The CAT scanner was an enormous step forward. Scans can show much greater detail than the normal X-ray tubes. There is no longer the problem of parts of the picture being completely hidden by bone shadows, and the machine can distinguish between very similar tissues; even the grey and white matter in the brain can be separated on CAT brain scans. In the early days it took machines nearly a minute to produce each picture, but with improvements in computer technology it is now possible to produce scans in 'real time'. Having produced a number of slices in one plane, the machine is able to re-calculate the results to construct new slices at right angles to the original ones. This has led to even greater ambitions, because the machines are still giving only two-dimensional pictures.

3-D
One way to produce three-dimensional scans is to store a number of individual slices in sequence on a holographic plate. Although holograms have been used for a few years by dentists, to keep records of their patients' mouths, they have been little used otherwise in medicine. One reason is that until recently it has only been possible to view holograms

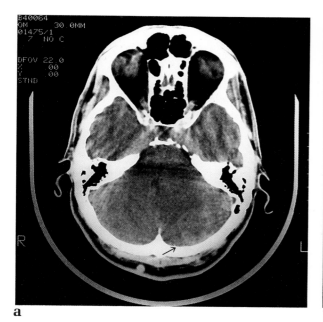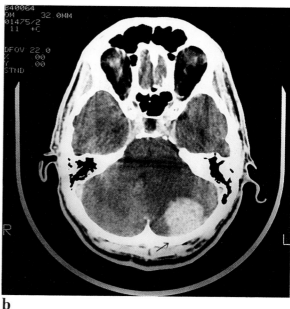

a

b

Two CAT scans of the same slice through the same head. In picture (a) a tumour is just visible; the signal is less regular on the left hand side at the back of the head. After the injection of a contrast medium (b) it is revealed much more clearly

in laser light, and in most hospitals lasers are not generally available. But now systems have been developed to look at holograms in ordinary light, so they could be just as easy to handle as ordinary X-rays. If sequences of scans were stored in this form it would be much easier for doctors to check, for instance, whether a tumour that is being treated is shrinking, growing, or standing still. At the moment it is often very difficult to judge.

An even more ambitious project at the University of Colorado Medical School aims to produce instant three-dimensional images on a screen while the patient is being scanned. It is really a computing problem; the information is there, and it is just a matter of putting it together. However, since it needs a computer capable of handling 500 million bits of information there is nothing simple about it. Also in America a system is being developed to use a sequence of stored images to create a 3-dimensional computer graphic on which a surgeon can try out a particular operating strategy – with images that change to show the result of any incision.

Nuclear medicine
In both the conventional X-ray and the CAT scan, the picture is produced by a signal from an X-ray source passing through the body and being partly absorbed. But there is another way. Radioactive isotopes, with half-lives ranging from a few seconds to a few days, can be injected into the body and then tracked with a camera that detects the gamma radiation they emit in order to see where they get to. One big advantage this method has over X-rays is that it can show not only the shape of an organ such as the heart, liver or kidney, but also whether its tissue is fully active or whether there are dead areas.

Say the object of a scan is to find out whether the right-hand kidney is functioning properly. The patient is given an injection of a radioactive isotope attached to a compound which will be transported within a few minutes to the kidney, where it will be eliminated from the blood. At the appropriate interval after the injection the kidney will be scanned by a gamma camera. A gamma camera can take a picture of all or part of its subject in much the same way as an ordinary camera does. Inside an ordinary camera, however, is film which is sensitive to light in the visible part of the spectrum, so the picture is the same as the one seen by the naked eye. In a gamma camera the film is replaced with a layer of sodium iodide crystals which 'see' only the much shorter wavelength gamma radiation. The crystal absorbs any gamma rays it receives and converts them into light scintillations which are displayed on a screen. Different intensities of radiation are shown as different colours, so the picture on the screen will be of a multicoloured contour map of the kidney with the most active areas shown in, say, blue, and areas of less activity in a range of other colours. In this way it is easy to detect which areas are much less active than they should be.

Radio-isotopes can be attached to a range of different substances depending on where the radiologist wants them to go. With some kinds of cancer a common place for secondary tumours to appear is in the bones. A radio-isotope can be attached to the appropriate molecule, which will depend on the origin of the tumour. This will be taken up by any tumour cells in the bone, and if the person is then scanned they will show up clearly.

One limitation of the images produced by the gamma camera is that they are, like the flat X-rays, two-dimensional pictures of a solid object rather than a slice. There is one type of radio-isotope that, using a computerized array of detectors, can produce an image similar to the CAT scan. This is the type of isotope that emits positrons.

BELOW LEFT Gamma camera image of the heart. The radioisotope is in the blood, and yellow areas reveal the strongest signal. This picture was taken when the left ventricle had contracted to pump the blood to the body. By taking a series of pictures the heart's action can be observed

BELOW RIGHT PET scans of brain showing blood flow (top) and metabolic activity (lower). The scans on the left are of the brain when the person being scanned had been in the dark for some time. Those on the right show the activity when the light was turned on and the eyes began to work. The highly active area (red-high; blue-low) at the back of the head is the part of the brain associated with sight

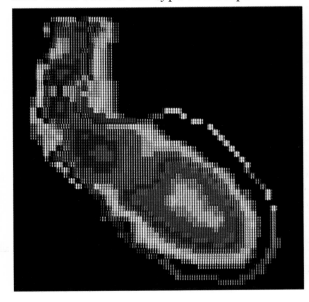

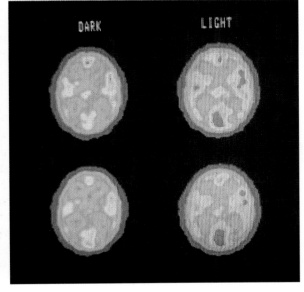

PET scanning

PET stands for positron emission tomography. The positron is a very peculiar particle, not a part of normal matter at all, but of antimatter; it is a positively charged electron. When a positron meets a normal negative electron the two particles react together violently and are annihilated in the process. The resulting energy is given off in the form of a pair of gamma rays travelling in opposite directions. Therefore the detection of a pair of such gamma rays indicates the presence, or rather the recent presence, of a positron; and because there are the two opposite rays it is possible to compute the precise point where the annihilation took place.

One of the principal uses of PET scanning to date has been in the study of metabolism, particularly in the brain. One of the isotopes that emits positrons is oxygen^{15}, and since oxygen is involved in providing the energy for metabolic activity a measure of oxygen consumption is also a measure of activity. Oxygen can be inhaled and its distribution in the body or brain measured by an array of gamma radiation detectors.

At the moment PET scanning is still very much a research tool, and its use is never likely to be widespread. The positron-emitting isotopes tend to be very short lived, no more than a matter of minutes, so PET scanning can only be done in the immediate vicinity of a cyclotron capable of creating the isotopes; and in Britain, for example, only a handful of hospitals have such a facility. The studies that have been done so far have been building up a picture of how normal tissues work. They have also given some useful information about the likely value of bypass operations to restore blood flow to areas of the brain damaged by stroke, and on identifying heart muscle that might recover following a heart attack. One possible future use is to check whether brain tissue transplants have 'taken' (see page 123).

There are two important challenges facing anyone who aims to develop new ways of looking through the body at what is going on inside. One is to provide new information, pictures that show the doctor something he could not see with any other system. The other important consideration is that the imaging system should not do any damage. Both X-rays and radio-isotopes involve ionizing radiation, rays that can be damaging to healthy tissue. In the early days the levels of radiation involved in diagnostic scanning worried nobody. It was not only in hospitals that such machines abounded. In the 1940s a visit to any well-equipped shoe shop was enlivened by a chance to watch the bones in your toes wiggling inside the new pair of shoes. By the end of the decade, however, people were becoming aware of the danger of any radiation, and the unnecessary machines were abandoned. The machines used in hospitals now produce less risk than earlier ones, and the dose from radio isotopes is small. But there are two systems which are thought to involve no risk at all: ultrasound and nuclear magnetic resonance.

Ultrasound

Ultrasound scanning is thought to be so safe that, unlike X-rays, it is regularly used for scanning pregnant women to check on the welfare of their babies. And the resolution of ultrasound pictures is now so good that it is used more and more in the diagnosis of disease although, with the exception of the baby scans, and possibly pictures of the heart, ultrasound pictures have the distinction of being highly informative to the expert and totally incomprehensible to any lay person who tries to make sense of them.

The picture is produced by a sort of sonar. In the scanner head, which is held in contact with the part of the body being scanned, is a piezoelectric crystal which vibrates as an electric current is fed to it, emitting a pulse like a sound wave but at a much higher frequency. (The frequency of audible sound is at about 20–20,000 Hz; an ultrasound scanner works at 3–7 MHz.) The pulse is transmitted straight into the body, and the crystal acts both as a transmitter and as a receiver, picking up the echo of each pulse as it is reflected back from the structures it meets.

An echo is created each time the pulse meets the interface between two different densities of tissue, like the surface of a bone or the edge of a lung. It can also detect much more subtle changes, such as the membrane surrounding an organ like the liver or kidney, or the wall of a blood vessel. The machine plots the returning echoes against time and produces a picture that is a slice straight down into the body.

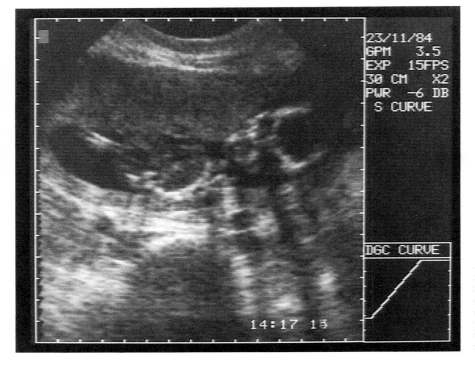

A baby scan, the most familiar use of ultrasound in medicine. By measuring the diameter of the head (the circle on the right of the picture) doctors can check that the baby is growing at the correct rate

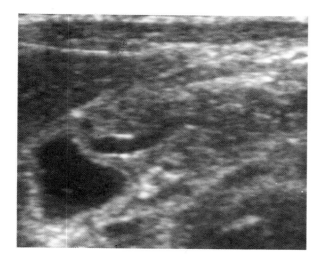 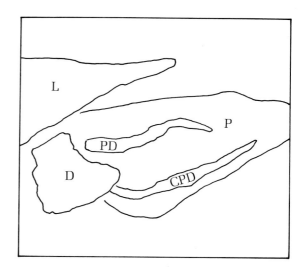

This picture tells the full story of why the patient is suffering abdominal pain — notoriously difficult to diagnose.

The pancreatic duct (PD) is in the wrong place, and its size shows that it is blocked. See below.

L = Liver
D = Duodenum
P = Pancreas
PD = Pancreatic duct
CPD = Correct position for pancreatic duct

Although ultrasound is regularly used to scan babies, in the past few years some people have expressed doubts about whether it is as safe as it has always been thought. The doubts were raised as a result of tests where subtle changes were produced in the chromosomes of cells exposed to ultrasound in culture. However, the levels of exposure in these tests were much more intense than in medical use, and doctors have pointed out that they have been using ultrasound for 20 years without any evidence at all that it causes damage. Ultrasound scanning has certainly opened up extraordinary possibilities.

Measurement of the diameter of the head can give early warning if the baby stops growing and needs help; but scans are also used to detect abnormalities, some of which can be put right. With an ultrasound picture to guide them doctors have been able to perform life-saving operations on unborn babies, draining fluid from a blocked bladder, or relieving pressure on the brain. In emergency, when a baby's heart stopped beating, it was even used to guide the doctor as he massaged the heart through the mother's abdomen and started it up again.

Sophisticated ultrasound scanners have many other uses, particularly to investigate diseases in the kidney, and in the area of the gall-bladder, bile ducts and pancreas, because it is the only type of scanner that can produce clear pictures of ducts in the liver without the use of injections of contrast. Some of the transmitter/detector probes are so small that they can be used inside the body, for instance to map tumours; and because ultrasound has no known side effects it is also the chosen method for research purposes, when the use of even the smallest dose of ionizing radiation would not be justified.

Doppler scanning

Doppler shift is the change in frequency of sound depending on whether the object producing the sound is travelling towards or away from the person who is hearing it. The classic example is the fire engine whose bell gets higher and higher pitched as it comes towards you and then climbs back down the scale again as it disappears into the distance. Ultrasound scanning can use the doppler shift to provide sometimes vital information about blood flow. If an ultrasound pulse strikes a moving substance, such as blood flowing through a vessel, then the frequency of the echo will be shifted just like the fire engine bell, depending on how fast the blood is flowing. This can often give early warning of the narrowing of a blood vessel, or of poor circulation in the limbs. It is particularly useful in checking the blood supply to a baby growing in the womb, because if the artery feeding it becomes narrowed the blood will be 'heard' speeding up.

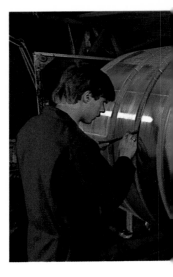

ABOVE Winding the magnetic coil for an MRI scanner. When fully wound it will contain 62 miles (100 kilometres) of wire

Magnetic resonance imaging

Originally known as nuclear magnetic resonance (the 'nuclear' was dropped because of its popular association with radioactivity), magnetic resonance imaging (MRI) is an entirely new way of producing pictures, based on the magnetic properties of atoms. Although magnetic resonance was used in the laboratory as early as the 1940s, it is only since 1980 that machines have been developed to look at the living body and produce pictures of its chemical structure.

The particles that make up the nucleus of the atom are protons and neutrons. Each of these particles is continuously spinning like a tiny top. The protons spin in the opposite direction to neutrons, so that when an atom has an equal number of each then the two types of spin cancel each other out. However, sometimes there are not an equal number of each, and then the spin creates a minute magnetic field, in the same way as the earth's spin creates the earth's magnetic field. In this situation, the nucleus can behave just like a tiny bar magnet, with a north and south pole. It is atoms of the 'odd' sort that are used in producing MRI pictures; a typical example is the hydrogen atom, which has just one nuclear particle, a proton, and is abundant throughout the body in all kinds of tissue.

BELOW Thermograph of a man with a cold nose and hands. White is hot, black is cold

Under normal circumstances, the hydrogen atoms in the body have their magnets aligned totally at random, which means they all cancel each other out, giving no magnetic effect. But when the body is put into a strong magnetic field then the atoms are all forced to line up in one of two ways: either parallel to the field or in the opposite direction to it, anti-parallel, as it is called. A nucleus that is sitting in the opposite direction to the field requires more energy; so it takes energy to switch a nucleus from parallel to anti-parallel, and a nucleus that switches from anti-parallel to the parallel state will give out energy. It is from this giving out of energy that the nuclear magnetic resonance picture is made.

The scanner itself is an enormous doughnut-shaped magnet, with a table through the middle on which the person being examined lies. To

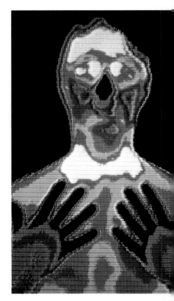

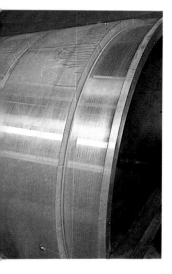

produce a powerful enough field (thousands of times stronger than the earth's) an electromagnet is used, usually with a superconducting coil, which is kept cold with liquid helium. Often the direction of the magnetic field is straight through the middle of the magnet, and then when the body is inside all the hydrogen nuclei will line up with the high energy ones facing the head, the low energy ones facing the toes. To create the picture, the operator wants to knock some of the lower energy protons into the high energy state, and then watch them dropping back. The extra energy to take the nuclei into the higher 'excited' state is supplied by waves beamed at the body from a radio frequency transmitter. When the signal is at precisely the right wavelength to resonate with the hydrogen nuclei they will absorb enough energy to knock them into

RIGHT Two magnetic resonance scans, taken from the side, of a vertical slice through the neck. The chin is on the left. The bright area on the right is a layer of fat, darkest areas are of fluid, and other tissues give various grey signals. The arrow points to the brain and spinal cord which is normal in the picture (a) but in picture (b) the cord is hollow and filled with fluid similar to that bathing the brain. Magnetic resonance is the only method of imaging that would reveal this

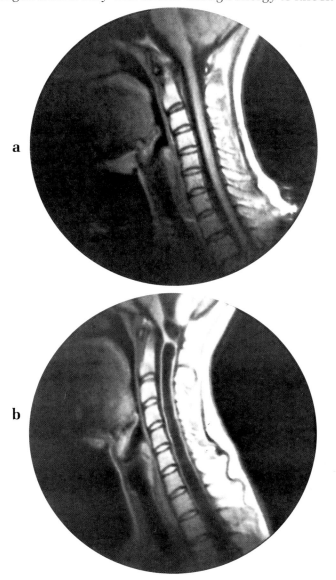

the anti-parallel position. Then when the pulse is turned off, the atoms will re-emit the energy as they drop back, and this re-emission can be picked up and analysed.

That signal can tell the scanner a great deal. The strength of the signal tells the machine how much hydrogen is there. In practice that often means how much water, but there is also hydrogen in fats and other molecules. The signals produced by the protons of hydrogen contained in water are different from the non-water hydrogen, so that provides another level of information. The time the hydrogen takes after the signal is turned off before it re-emits the energy it has absorbed is also very important, because this too can indicate what type of molecule the hydrogen is bound in. Yet more information is gleaned from a measurement of the rate at which the return to normal happened.

Having made all the measurements, the machine combines them to give a picture of the area it is looking at, and this picture can often give information that is not available from even the best CAT scan. One great advantage of MRI is that it does not rely on only one factor (X-rays, for instance, compare only the density of tissues), and this makes it more flexible. It is the only method discovered so far of producing pictures that show abnormalities in the brain and nerves, of the kind that cause multiple sclerosis. This means that it can be used not only to diagnose the disease, but also to give information about the usefulness of treatments. This is very valuable, because the course of the disease is so unpredictable that it is terribly difficult to tell whether a treatment is any use at all. It is also hoped that MRI will be helpful in producing information about the heart muscle and blood flow in the heart, and its ability to distinguish between types of tissue mean it may even be possible to use the scanners to tell whether of not a tumour is cancerous.

Magnetic resonance is not only used for producing pictures. With different computer software, the machine can be used to make measurements of biochemical processes taking place in living tissue. Phosphorus is another atom with an odd number of nuclear particles (31) and this can be examined instead of hydrogen. Phosphorus is an important constituent of ATP (adenosine triphosphate), the chemical involved in the delivery of energy for use in muscles and other tissues, and MRI biochemical measurements have already suggested ways of treating muscle problems. Just how useful this type of investigation may be is not yet known, because in most areas researchers are still at the stage of establishing what is normal, and only then will it be possible to recognize and interpret abnormalities.

One of the advantages of the nuclear magnetic resonance system is that no ionizing radiation is involved. There is no known ill effect from subjecting a body to this type of magnetic field, and the radio waves are at frequencies that are regularly used for normal shortwave transmission; such radiation is passing through us all the time. So it is very safe for the patient, but for the operator it has to be treated with care. The power of the magnetic field is so great that it is very dangerous to take any ferrous metal objects into the scanner room. A spanner can be turned into a lethal projectile if the magnetic field once gets hold of it. It also has less dangerous, but rather embarrassing, habits like wiping all the information off magnetic tapes and credit cards.

Heat and light

Nuclear magnetic resonance is the most sophisticated concept of scanning so far, but simpler forms of radiation, like heat and light, have their uses. Scanners making use of a mixture of red and infra-red light are being tested on screening programmes for breast cancer. Since the most usual scanning technique for this involves X-rays, this non-ionizing light would be preferable if it proves to be as reliable.

Many illnesses, like rheumatoid arthritis, diseases of arteries and veins, and some cancers produce hot or cold spots in the body which are often detectable on the skin. It is useful to be able to measure them accurately, not only for diagnosis, but particularly to check whether treatment is producing results. Cameras using infra-red sensors have been developed that can detect hot spots with temperature differences as little as one-twentieth of a degree C.

Infra-red sensors can pick up heat from the skin, but if the source of the heat is not very near the surface it may not reach the skin to be detected. However, the hot spot will be producing radiation not only in the infra-red part of the spectrum, but also in the microwave, and this radiation is much more penetrating, so it is more likely to reach the surface. Instruments have been developed to detect this microwave radiation, and they are now undergoing tests. The hope of the developers is that the instruments may be useful in detecting a number of diseases, but once again one of their targets is early breast cancer. It has never been proved that early detection of breast cancer gives a better chance of survival, but it is reasonable to assume that it does; and, of course, all these heat cameras have the advantage that they must be totally safe, since all they do is pick up existing signals.

All of these scanners are designed to give a view inside the body, through layers that are not transparent to normal eyes. But sometimes it is difficult to see an object which is completely visible. Our eyes do not give us really good three-dimensional vision, and sometimes that is a problem. Pictures like that on the left are designed to overcome this problem. It is a contour map, made by shining light on to the body from two standard 35 mm slide projectors, one on each side. In front of each projector is a grid, which allows the light through only in very fine lines, and this produces the contour pattern. It is not quite as simple as that, because special lenses are needed to reduce the distortion that would be caused by the spread of the projector's beam. With the help of a contour map like this it is very easy to see what happens when the child breathes in: a distortion that might easily be missed by the naked eye.

An 11 year-old boy takes a deep breath, and the contour map clearly reveals his displaced rib

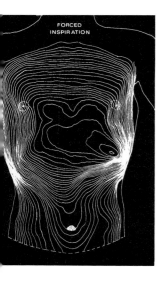

FORCED INSPIRATION

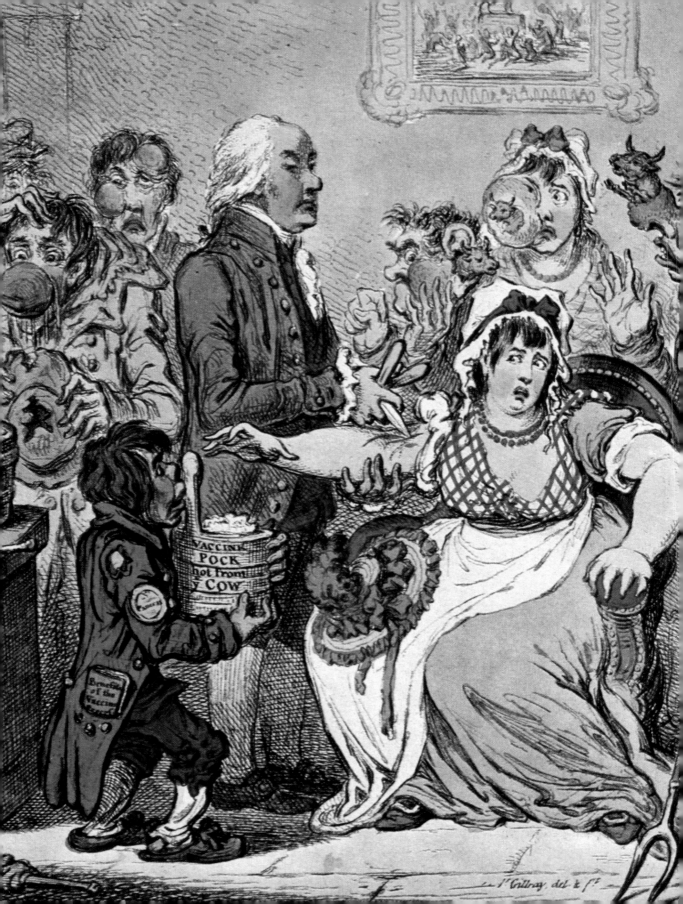

CHAPTER TWO

Self-Defence

OPPOSITE The reaction of the cartoonist James Gillray to the idea of vaccination

The human race would have died out long before the birth of scientific medicine had it not been for the immune system. In fact we could never have developed in the first place, surrounded as we are by a mass of hostile forces: viruses, bacteria, fungal infections, and larger organisms like those causing many tropical diseases, not to mention the continuous bombardment of cosmic rays. The immune system has kept man as a species one step ahead of all these enemies. Medicine's task has been to help the individual members of the species whose immune system is not working efficiently, and the earliest real successes in treating infectious disease were achieved not with drugs but by enhancing natural immunity. Vaccination and other forms of immunization are designed to arm the body's own defence mechanism, and they were developed long before there was any idea of how they worked. A much better understanding of the immune system is now laying the foundation of what could be the next revolution in the treatment of infectious disease, cancer and a range of other ills.

The first person who produced any real information on the workings of the immune system was the Russian biologist Ilya Mechnikov, who made his observations in 1882 – not in humans but in starfish. He was watching some transparent starfish larvae under his microscope one day when he noticed mobile cells swimming about inside the larvae, and it occurred to him that cells like those might in some way be involved in defending the animal against invaders. To try out his theory he collected some rose thorns from the garden and inserted them under the skin of some of the larvae. Then he waited to see what would happen, and sure enough his mobile cells surrounded the rose thorns, like ants attacking a foreign invader of the colony. He repeated the experiment using bacteria instead of thorns, and saw the same thing happening. This was the first piece of the picture that is gradually building up of the immune system.

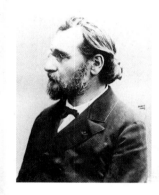

ABOVE Ilya Mechnikov, the founder of immunology

Mechnikov had a very simple theory of how the system works, and we now know it is really extremely complicated. There are many different types of defence cell, and many details of their various roles, and the mechanism that controls them, are still eluding scientists. But it is only by understanding these mechanisms that we have any real hope of dealing effectively with such massive problems as rheumatoid arthritis, some diabetes and multiple sclerosis, as well as cancer and the more obviously connected diseases like viral infections and the recently described disease AIDS. All of these diseases result from the immune system losing control of the situation in some way that is still obscure. However, a great deal has already been discovered.

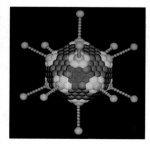

BELOW Molecular computer graphic of adenovirus, the cause of the common cold

The whole system depends on the fact that it is possible to recognize the difference between the body's own cells and the cells of an invader. Every living thing, whether it is a bacterium or virus or single human cell, carries on its coat complicated protein (or occasionally carbohydrate) molecules, called antigens, which mark it out as an individual, and the immune system learns to recognize all the different antigens that belong to itself. Any unfamiliar protein it encounters is therefore obviously an enemy and must be dealt with as such. (This can be unfortunate when the unfamiliar protein is part of a transplanted organ, and it would be very useful to have some way of telling the body clearly that this antigen, although unfamiliar, is nevertheless friendly.) Not only do the invading organisms carry foreign markings themselves, but when one of the body's own cells is invaded by a virus, or when it undergoes the sort of changes that could lead to a cancer, then it too may begin to develop new proteins on its surface which should mark it out as unfriendly.

The actual work of recognizing and repelling invaders is done by the white cells of the blood, also known as leucocytes. There are many different kinds of leucocyte, all with their separate roles, but between them they have three ways of handling invaders: swallowing them, attacking with chemicals and attacking with antibodies.

First there are the phagocytes. The name comes from the Greek *phagein* meaning 'eat', and their role is to swallow up and dispose tidily of any invaders or damaged cells in the body. Some are able to recognize and deal with invaders without help, but some need assistance from one of the other types of cell, the lymphocytes.

B-lymphocytes and T-lymphocytes both originate from cells in the bone marrow. They are present not only in the blood but also, as their name implies, in the lymph, the clear fluid that surrounds all the cells, and carries nutrients from the blood vessels to the cells and returns waste products. Often invading bacteria that find their way into the body through a cut are destroyed in the lymph system before they ever reach the blood vessels.

Although B-lymphocytes and T-lymphocytes look exactly the same, they work in entirely different ways. B-lymphocytes are responsible for recognizing invading organisms, or the poisonous substances such organisms often produce, and for making antibodies to them. Antibodies are large, complicated molecules specially designed to fit precisely on to the identifying proteins on the surface of the invaders. These antibodies are not usually able to kill the invaders themselves. What they do is start off a process in which the organism is actually destroyed by a series of chemical reactions which are known all together as complement. In the beginning it was thought that complement was just one chemical substance, but now it is known that it is a series of reactions in no fewer than nine stages.

T-lymphocytes play a quite different role, and have developed in a different way from the B-cells. They are called T-cells because they have been 'educated' in the thymus gland. The 'education' is thought to involve learning how to tell the difference between self and non-self, although nobody is quite sure how it operates. The T-cells seem to be in command of the whole immune process, and they exercise their control

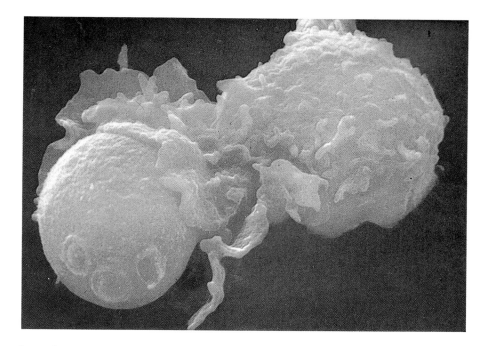

Scanning electron micrograph shows a white cell swallowing up a yeast cell

by releasing a variety of chemical signals, which can call other cells to the scene or tell them to multiply. Like the B-cells they can recognize foreign proteins, but they do not make antibody. Instead they play a variety of specialist roles. They can become killer cells, which attack with chemicals; they can be T-helper cells, which play an important part in the activity of both B-cells and killer cells; or they can call up reinforcements of cells which will turn into highly active phagocytes, sometimes known as 'angry' phagocytes. Another extremely important function of T-cells is that of the T-suppressor cell, which turns the activity off when it is no longer needed. The relative importance of all the different types of cell in the defence of the body varies depending on the type of attack, and whether it comes from a virus, a bacterium or a cancer. Most of the ways that medicine has developed for harnessing the immune system make use of the more specific of the defence cells, the B-lymphocytes and T-lymphocytes.

The first time the body is attacked by a particular intruder, for example a virus, it calls up its first line of defence, both phagocytes and cells called natural killers which attack with chemicals. But the more effective specific defenders, the B-cells and T-cells, are unable to respond immediately. It may take a number of days for a group of cells to be found and prepared to handle that particular invader. Nobody is quite sure how this is done, but it is thought that a sample of the invader is taken to the nearest lymph gland and it is there that the programming and multiplying of the B-cells and T-cells takes place. During those days, the virus has a chance to multiply and gain a strong hold. However, once that group of B-cells and T-cells has been produced, some representatives of the group will carry on circulating in the body indefinitely, ready to attack instantly if that intruder ever appears again. So an individual is very unlikely to suffer the same disease twice.

Vaccination

The idea of vaccination is to give a person's B- and T-cells a chance to arm themselves against an organism without giving him the disease that organism normally causes. We know now that the reason why smallpox vaccination worked was that the cowpox virus, which was harmless to humans, carried some antigens identical to smallpox, so that the immune cells could be armed against smallpox simply by meeting the cowpox virus. Later types of immunization to be developed use the real organism that causes a disease, but after weakening it or even killing it first. Louis Pasteur weakened his viruses by exposing them to the air; other methods involve growing them in the laboratory over and over again, or treating them with heat or chemicals.

Now we know that a vaccine does not depend for its effect on introducing the immune system to the whole organism, but really to the antigens on its surface, other ways of developing new vaccines are being tried which do not rely simply on killing or weakening viruses. With the development of genetic engineering it is possible to concentrate on putting into vaccines only the parts of the viruses that are essential.

Hepatitis B is an extremely serious viral disease affecting the liver. It has mainly hit the headlines in the past when it has spread in kidney dialysis units or among hospital workers because of contact with infected blood. It is incurable, often fatal, and can cause liver cancer, so a vaccine against hepatitis B is also a vaccine against cancer. One became available some years ago, but it was scarce and expensive because it had to be made from the blood of immune individuals. To make a satisfactory vaccine, however, all that is needed is the surface protein of the virus, and the part of the hepatitis B genetic material that makes the important antigen has been isolated. This has been transferred into yeast cells, and when grown in a fermenter these yeast cells make large quantities of the protein, without making the parts of the virus that do all the damage. Early tests suggest that this yeast-made hepatitis B protein will produce an immunity that is just as good as the earlier vaccine – and it should be much cheaper, an important consideration in a disease which is widespread in the developing world.

Diseases like cholera which cause disastrous diarrhoea result in 10 million deaths every year. Although a cholera vaccine has been available for many years, its effect lasts for a very short time: only six months or so. This means that it has really only been any use to travellers visiting areas where the disease is common. People who live there have only been able to obtain immunity by suffering and surviving the disease, and many fail to survive.

The cholera bacterium causes its symptoms by producing a poisonous protein which attacks the gut wall, and given time the immune system is able to make antibodies to this poison, or toxin, just as it can against a bacterium or virus. It has now been shown that it is just one small section of the toxin molecule that does all the damage, and when

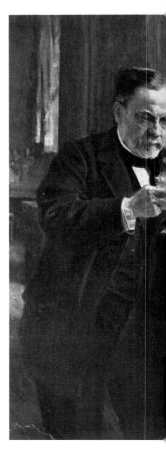

Louis Pasteur was the first man to develop a human vaccine from a live virus. He is here shown holding a flask containing the spinal cord of a rabbit in which he weakened the rabies virus

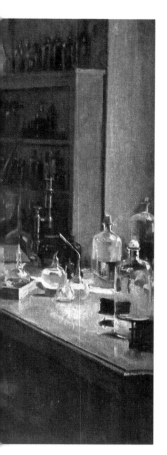

this section is removed the toxin will still provoke the body into making antibodies. More to the point, these antibodies are effective not only against the harmless modified protein, but also against the deadly intact protein. The toxin itself can be modified chemically, but some experts think a much more effective vaccine would be one made with the whole cholera organism, but with its genetic material changed so that it produces only the harmless version of the poison molecule. Such a vaccine has been produced and it gave excellent immunity. However, it also produced a few side effects, so more work needs to be done before it is released.

There are vaccines available now to protect against many of the serious diseases of the developed world. Third World diseases are still presenting problems, partly because commercial pressures to produce vaccines have not been so great, but also because the organisms that cause the diseases have life cycles that make them much more difficult to attack.

Malaria is mainly a disease of the Third World, although it is certainly seen elsewhere. In Britain about 1500 cases occur a year, mainly in people returning from abroad, and it can result in death even when good medical treatment is available. The need to develop a malaria vaccine has become more urgent in recent years because of two developments. The most serious type of malaria is caused by an organism called *Plasmodium falciparum*, and in many parts of the world this is resistant to the most commonly used drug. The second development concerns the way the disease is spread. Malaria is carried by mosquitoes, and at one time there were high hopes that a chemical attack on them with DDT and other insecticides might wipe them out. Now DDT is out of favour because of its long-term environmental dangers, and other insecticides have proved much less effective.

The problem about developing a vaccine against malaria is that, in common with many other tropical diseases, the organism that causes it has a complicated life cycle. The parasite is born in the mosquito. When the mosquito bites a human being it injects its saliva, and with it the malaria organism in a form called a sporozoite. This travels immediately to the liver, and in the cells of the liver the organism begins changes that result in a new form, called a merozoite. Returned from the liver to the bloodstream, some of the creatures change yet again into a stage called a gametocyte before being sucked out in a blood meal by a new mosquito, where it will mate and produce large numbers of new sporozoites. In each of these different forms the organism has quite different antigens on its coat. So an immune cell armed against one stage would be helpless against another.

The easiest stage to make a vaccine against would be the first, the sporozoite, because the proteins involved are very simple ones, and in fact they have been made in quantities. But there are doubts about whether a vaccine containing only this antigen would be effective,

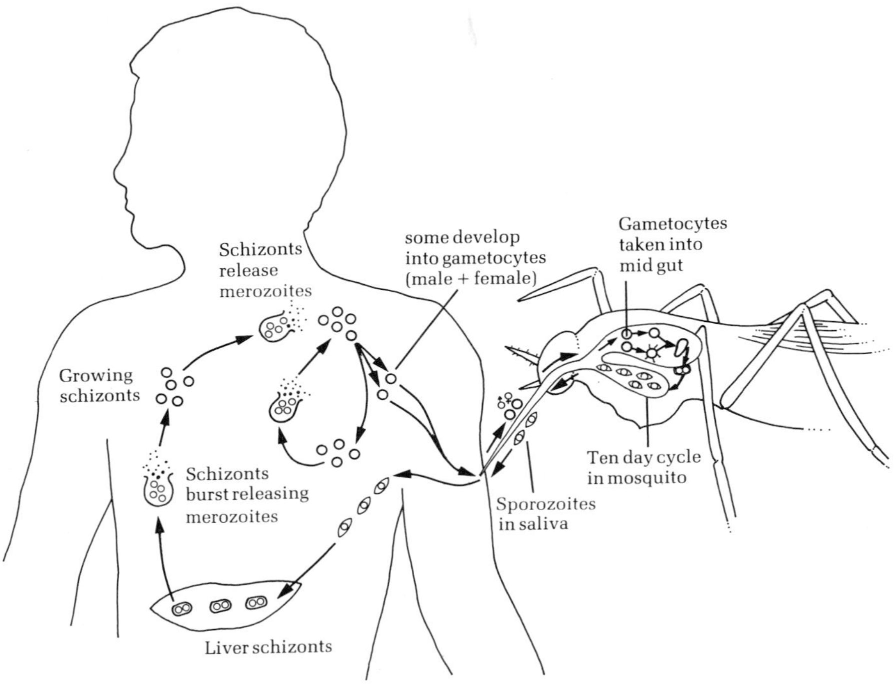

The life cycle of the organism that causes malaria

Schizonts release merozoites

some develop into gametocytes (male + female)

Gametocytes taken into mid gut

Growing schizonts

Schizonts burst releasing merozoites

Ten day cycle in mosquito

Sporozoites in saliva

Liver schizonts

because the malaria organism spends only a very short time, a matter of minutes, in this form before it enters a liver cell. It will emerge into the bloodstream again disguised so that the 'armed' immune system will not recognize it.

One team of researchers have found the material for a potential vaccine which works at the other end of the organism's stay in its human host. They have found a way of producing an antibody to the gametocyte, which makes the organism incapable of reproducing. However, that approach has the disadvantage that while it would possibly prevent the spread of disease in the long term there is very little motivation for an individual to present himself for a shot of this vaccine, since it will do nothing to preserve him personally from the effects of the disease, which are produced by the parasite in its earlier stages.

The important target is obviously the middle stage, which is more difficult because the organism is more complicated. So yet another team of researchers have been looking in the blood of immune individuals in parts of the world where the disease is common, to see what antibodies they have produced to give them their protection against the parasite. The researchers have examined a number of these antibodies now, although they have not so far managed to find a really good candidate from which they might make a vaccine.

In the long term what scientists would really like to do is to make a single vaccine that could cover all the stages of the disease. To do so they plan to use the oldest and the newest tools of the immunologists. The oldest is the vaccinia virus, the type of virus Edward Jenner used to vaccinate against smallpox. The newest is the technique of genetic engineering.

To make the multi-purpose malaria vaccine, the genetic engineers would need to start not with the antigens that will induce the invaded body to produce antibodies, but with the various pieces of the malaria parasite's genetic material that carry the blueprint for those antigens. Each of these genes, one or two for each stage of the parasite's life cycle, would then be 'stitched' into the genetic material of a vaccinia virus, an accommodating creature which is quite willing to carry other organisms' genes around. A virus modified in this way would incorporate malaria-type proteins in its coat, so when used as a vaccine it should provoke the production of a range of malaria antibodies. This technique has already been tried out with hepatitis B antigens, as an alternative to growing them in yeast cells, and it has been tested successfully, at least in animals.

In fact it seems possible that this type of vaccine might be directed at more than one disease. Polyvalent vaccines, as they are called, might well be made containing not only all the stages of the malaria parasite, but also genes for antigens connected with other diseases that are prevalent in the same area: a truly multi-purpose vaccine.

Flu
One thing that has infuriated immunologists for a long time is the difficulty of creating a vaccine for influenza. It is almost as maddening as the impossibility of curing the common cold. In most cases flu is not a dangerous disease, but in the weak or the elderly, or in people who also have other diseases, it can be fatal. Even when it is not fatal it means a week or so away from work, and most people take much longer to recover fully from a bad attack, so it is well worth preventing. But although vaccines have been developed they are not very satisfactory.

The problem with the flu virus is not that it has a complicated life cycle like malaria, but that there are a whole family of viruses, and each separate strain carries a set of antigens that are different from the others. So a vaccine prepared to cope with one strain will give the body no help at all in recovering from infection with a different one. Not only is there the difficulty of predicting which particular variety of flu will strike in a given year, but the virus has the ability to change its coat, altering the tell-tale proteins enough to fool the immune system into taking it as new and starting again from scratch.

Researchers believe the solution to this may be to look for a vaccine that will produce a different type of immunity: not B-cell immunity but T-cell. Just as the B-cells that produce antibodies have the ability to recognize and remember foreign proteins, so do the T-cells. However, T-cells only act against foreign proteins when they meet them in conjunction with particular 'self' proteins on the surface of an infected cell. When a virus has entered a cell and taken control of it, the cell will build virus proteins into its own outer membrane. When that has happened the T-cell can encounter the viral protein in the right circumstances to allow it to fix onto the cell and attack with its armoury of destructive chemicals.

Whereas the protein coats of flu viruses differ from strain to strain, the researchers think that some of these proteins incorporated into the cell walls are more consistent, so by aiming at this type of immune reaction it should be possible to arm the body against more than one strain at a time. But the killed flu viruses used in vaccines at the moment do not allow the virus to incorporate its genes and so build proteins into the cell membrane, so the T-lymphocytes are never armed against it.

The scientists using this approach plan to work out which of the eight genes of the virus are responsible for these proteins. Then, just like the malaria workers, they might possibly use the vaccinia virus to carry the gene into the cells, so that the T-lymphocytes may in a very real sense 'read, mark and learn' it.

Vaccination is a way of pre-arming the immune system to prevent a disease from taking hold; the body becomes active in its own defence. But except in the case of a slowly incubating disease like rabies, vaccination has no value once an individual has been infected with an organism. Then the immune system needs a different kind of help, a supply of antibodies produced by another person (or animal). Before the development of a vaccine, diphtheria was a common disease among children and caused many horrible deaths. The bacterium responsible for the disease produced a poison, or toxin, which spread throughout the whole body and it was with an antibody to this that the first treatment of an infectious disease with immune serum was performed. The antibodies were grown in the blood of horses, which were chosen because they were large enough to provide large quantities of serum without ill effects. The animals were inoculated with the disease at intervals over a month to allow the antibodies to build up in their blood. Then the blood was taken and purified to remove all the cells and as much of the unwanted protein as was possible, and then injected into the affected child. The treatment was successful and was used widely. Fortunately diphtheria is now a rare disease, but tetanus antitoxin is still commonly used, as are antibodies to the poisons contained in snakebite. Antiserum is also used, but this time to the whole organism, in virus diseases like Lassa fever which are so rare in developed countries that none of us has a chance to build up immunity.

Antibodies and monoclonal antibodies
In both vaccines and antitoxins, antibodies are used more or less as nature intended. But the ability of an antibody to distinguish between molecules that are indistinguishable by any other means has opened up possibilities for other uses. Work with antibodies and monoclonal antibodies promises to lead to the next medical 'revolution'.

The immune systems of all higher animals are programmed to make antibodies to any foreign protein they meet. This may be an infectious organism or an antitoxin, but it may just as well be cells or proteins from another animal. It has been calculated that a mouse's B-cells have the ability to make a million different antibodies. How this capacity is built into the animal's genes is still partly a mystery, but whether or not that mouse, or its ancestors, have ever met the antigen before, its immune system is still able to raise a line of B-lymphocytes to make antibody to any newly encountered protein. In medical practice animal immune systems are used to raise antibodies to specific types of human tissue. These antibodies can be recovered from the blood and used in exceedingly sensitive tests.

There is a condition called Cushing's disease in which a person's blood chemistry becomes badly upset, his muscles begin to waste and he becomes very weak and susceptible to infection. To make sure that the illness is in fact Cushing's disease it is important to check whether the level of a hormone called ACTH (adreno-corticotrophic hormone) is raised. Hormones like this appear in the blood in minute quantities; what is more they are chemically very similar to other hormones, and with normal chemical techniques it is virtually impossible to detect raised levels. But a test using antibodies can detect a few parts in a thousand million.

To make antibody for the test an animal, say a rabbit, is injected with a quantity of ACTH. The rabbit will begin to make antibodies to the hormone, and after a few weeks a quantity of the animal's blood is taken and the antibody is extracted and purified. This becomes the laboratory's standard preparation for measuring ACTH levels. A patient comes in with a possible hormone abnormality and gives a blood sample. The hormone will be in the serum – what is left of the blood after the red cells, white cells and clotting agents have been removed – so first of all these are separated out and, as Mrs Beeton used to say, discarded. A measured amount of the rabbit antibody is put into a test tube, together with the sample to be tested, and also a known amount of ACTH from another source that has been made radioactive. The rabbit antibodies will stick to the two different types of ACTH in the same proportion as they are present in the mixture. So if 80 per cent of the antibody sticks to radioactive ACTH and only 20 per cent to cold (non-radioactive), then that means that the amount of radioactive hormone (which is known) is four times as great as the amount in the serum being tested.

To check how much of each type of ACTH is bound to antibody, the antigen/antibody complexes are clumped together (this can be done with a different type of antibody) and removed from the mixture, and the level of bound radioactivity is counted. If the counts are high it must mean that most of the radioactive hormone has been able to bind to the antibody; there can have been very little in the test sample to compete with it for 'partners'. If the counts are low it means that the competition was fierce, so there was a lot of the hormone in the test sample.

Two T-killer cells attacking an influenza infected cell

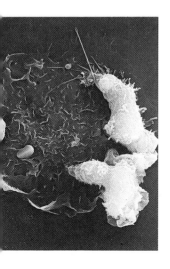

These tests can be used to make extremely accurate measurements of the levels of hormones of various kinds, not only ACTH. In fact in the case of Cushing's disease the hormone may be even more helpful. ACTH is normally made by the pituitary, a gland situated in the middle of the head, just below the brain. If the level of ACTH in the blood is raised the most likely reason is that there is a tumour in the pituitary (a benign one, not a cancer). This may show on a CAT scan, but it may not, and there is another possible explanation: occasionally ACTH is produced by a tumour somewhere else in the body. When it is suspected that this is the case, a number of blood samples can be taken from different blood vessels and the hormone levels checked. When they are compared it is clear which vein has the highest level and is therefore closest downstream of the tumour. This may be the only way of finding the tumour if it is only a few millimetres across and hidden, for instance, in the middle of a lobe of the lung.

Antibody tests of this sort can be developed to check the level of any individual protein – with one proviso. The process has to begin with a pure sample of the relevant protein, and the only easy way to separate out individual hormones is with antibodies. At the beginning of the chain somebody has to purify the protein the hard way. This is usually done by separating out the molecules according to their molecular weight on gradient columns. One recently isolated protein is a small chemical produced in the brain to carry a message to the pituitary, telling it to produce a hormone which in its turn will instruct the thyroid gland to secrete yet another hormone (the system is like that). This protein is made in such small quantities that the scientist who isolated it used material from the brains of two million sheep which he separated out on a gradient column two storeys high.

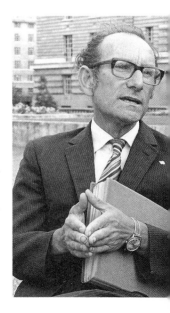

Dr Cesar Milstein developer, with Georges Koehler, of the monoclonal antibody

There are two main limitations in antibodies made in the traditional way for medical use. The first is that they come in such immense variety that it is extremely difficult, if not impossible, to purify them to such a degree that they behave consistently. Even a single protein may have a number of sites on its surface for which antibodies can be made, so when it is injected into an animal the creature's immune system will produce a range of antibodies, and these will be mixed with any other antibodies it has in its blood at that time. The second problem is that supplies may be limited. Some of the rarer antibodies may be held by only one organization in a country, in fact they may all come from one animal, and when that animal dies then the tests that depend on accurate measurements may need calibrating all over again. A technique developed by a team in Cambridge, which won them a share in the 1984 Nobel Prize for Medicine, overcame both of these problems at once. This is the technique for making monoclonal antibodies.

Monoclonal antibodies

A monoclonal antibody (MCA) is an antibody that is made in tissue culture by a population of cells all of which are descended from one individual cell, and all of which should therefore be identical. Antibodies are only made by B-lymphocytes, and one particular B-lymphocyte can make only one type of antibody. So all the antibodies from the descendant of one B-lymphocyte should be identical.

The reason why development of this technique merited a Nobel Prize was that it was extremely difficult to persuade B-lymphocytes to grow outside the body, and success in doing so has opened up immense possibilities to medicine, although before these can be realized there are formidable obstacles to be overcome.

Most normal adult animal cells do not grow happily in tissue culture; however good the conditions in which they are being cultured they will die after just a very few divisions. Cancer cells, on the other hand, will continue to grow and divide vigorously as long as they have sufficient nutrient and the right circumstances. (It is precisely this ability that enables a cancer to do the damage it does.) The team who developed the monoclonal antibody technique found a way of combining the immortality of the cancer cell with the antibody-producing ability of the B-lymphocyte.

The process starts in the same way as in traditional antibody production by injecting an animal with an antigen, and leaving it to produce B-lymphocytes programmed to make the appropriate antibody. Then they collect B-cells either from the blood of the animal, or more often from the spleen or one of the lymph glands, and mix them with some cells from a cancer of the lymphocytes called myeloma. (If the B-cells come from a mouse, so should the cancer.) The cells are mixed together in a solution of chemicals, among them polyethylene glycol, which reduces the surface tension round the cells and allows them to come into intimate contact, and during this process some of the cells will fuse together making composite B-lymphocyte/cancer cells called hybridomas. The mixture now contains three types of cell – cancer cells, B-lymphocytes and hybridomas – and these are put into a new culture medium in which the unfused cancer cells will be unable to grow, the unfused B-cells will die anyway, and so the only cells that survive will be the mixed ones, the hybridomas.

Of course, the lymphocytes taken from the animal will be a mixture, producing a large range of antibodies, all but a very few of which will have nothing to do with the important antigen. (The mouse, remember, can make a million different antibodies.) So the hybrid cells, too, will be producing a variety of different antibodies. The cells have to be spread out so that each one is growing on its own. Then they can be left to grow, and can be checked to see what they are producing. There are a variety of techniques for growing and sorting the cells, but they are all laborious and it can take years to find an important antibody. Once found, it can be a very valuable property. Genetic engineering companies can make fortunes out of individual monoclonal antibodies that are useful in

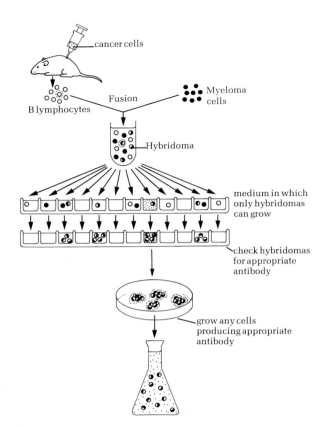

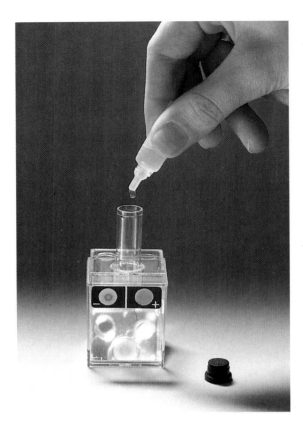

ABOVE LEFT Making a
monocolonal antibody
ABOVE RIGHT A pregnancy
test kit. One of the earliest
large scale uses of a
monoclonal antibody

frequently performed tests, because once a population of cells is established it can be grown on a large scale making very big quantities of the antibody very easily.

For some time now monoclonal antibodies have been used in pregnancy test kits, where they detect hormone levels and indicate the presence of a pregnancy by producing a colour change. Another cell line that was developed early in the hunt produced an antibody to digitalis, a drug that many people take for heart disease. Because one person's body may react to this drug in a different way from another's, it is very difficult to work out the correct dosage. In some people digitalis can build up in the blood, and then it becomes very dangerous. The antibody can be used not only to measure the level of drug in the blood; it also acts as an antidote, blocking the poisonous activity of the drug if it does reach too high a level.

As more different MCAs are found they will be able to detect much finer differences between groups of cells than are possible otherwise, and produce accurate measurements of hormones, enzymes and other biological molecules. In various centres they are being used or tried out as a possible new means of assessing damage in heart attack, brain injury or injury to other organs, to give early warning of the threat of coronary thrombosis, and to produce an easy test of thyroid disorders. So that their presence can be detected, they can be labelled radioactively or used to precipitate a colour change, or tagged with a chemical that will fluoresce in ultraviolet light. The last method of labelling is very useful, because this fluorescence can be used in mechanized cell sorters. A stream of cells can be passed through a detector and each cell directed to right or left into separate collectors depending on whether or not it fluoresces.

Blood groups

The ABO blood groups are based on differences in antigens on the red cells. The reason why matched blood has to be used for transfusion is that otherwise the immune system of the recipient will attack the newly arrived red cells and break them open. But some variation is possible as long as it is in the right direction. So far as the ABO antigens are concerned, owners of group O blood have non-antigenic red cells; there are no antigens on the surface of the cells that will cause them to be attacked by any other human immune system. Thus group O blood can be given to anyone. Group A blood has a particular antigen, so is only suitable for other As or ABs, both of whom will have immune systems programmed to accept the A antigen as self. Group B will have blood suitable for other Bs and ABs. AB blood is only acceptable to other ABs. The 'disadvantaged' group are the Os, whose blood can be taken for anyone, but who have to find another group O person when they are in need of a transfusion. The British National Blood Transfusion Service does virtually all of its basic blood grouping now with the aid of MCAs, because antibodies exist for both the A and B antigens and for the rhesus factor which is another antigenic difference between individuals. Another MCA has been developed to make recipients of blood transfusions safer by checking donor blood for the presence of the dangerous virus hepatitis B.

Transplants

Finding compatible blood donors is much easier than finding transplant donors because the variability of antigens on red cells is extremely small compared with that on white cells and other tissues. One set of variables in tissue is known as the HLA system (histocompatibility leucocyte antigens), called that because they were first found on leucocytes, but they also occur on most other cells. Tissue typing, to find pairs of people between whom a transplant might be possible, involves discovering which of a possible range of HLAs each individual carries. The complicated system for checking these at the moment could be very much simplified if monoclonal antibodies could be made for all the various antigens in this system. There are some MCAs that are useful in tissue typing, but finding others is proving difficult, partly because of the fact that the cells that make the antibodies come from animals. When given HLA molecules to make antibodies against, a mouse or rat is more likely to make an antibody against the part of the molecule that says 'human' rather than the part which distinguishes between the different tissue types. If the hybrid cells for producing the antibodies could be made from human lymphocytes and cancer cells, then they would be more likely to make useful antibodies, but human hybrid cells are proving even more difficult to make than animal ones, and so far they do not grow so well or so quickly.

Human cells would not only be more likely to produce antibodies that could distinguish between different tissue types, they would also be much safer. Some of the uses now being developed involve not a test on a blood sample, but injection of antibody into the living person – and there is a definite danger that when animal-made antibodies are injected into the blood they can clump together, causing a condition called serum sickness, or provoke a violent, even lethal, immune reaction. Antibodies made from human cells would be much less likely to cause either of these problems.

It is in the diagnosis and treatment of cancer in particular that it may in the future be important to be able to inject large amounts of antibody. There is no question that the proteins in the cell membrane change when a cell becomes cancerous, and that these changes should be enough to alert the immune system to the fact that something is wrong, although for some unknown reason the immune system fails to destroy the malignant cell. Not only do the proteins on the cell surface change, but these proteins are also shed into the bloodstream, and ought to be detectable there. In fact in theory it should be possible to create a range of cancer test kits much like the pregnancy ones. Yet although numerous researchers have been hunting for special cancer antigens in the ten years since monoclonal antibodies became possible, not a single one has been found. A number of proteins have been found that are at abnormally high levels in people with various types of tumour like cancers of the colon, ovaries, uterus, cervix, prostate, lungs and liver. But all of these antigens also appear at low levels in healthy individuals, and at intermediate levels in smokers and sufferers from a variety of non-malignant diseases. However the search for specific antigens goes on because they could lead to so many interesting possibilities.

Although the MCAs existing at the moment are not exclusively associated with cancer cells, they are so much more prevalent in cancer cells that they are already being used to confirm the presence of the condition, and also to help to indicate the precise position and size of the tumour.

Antibodies that have a strong affinity for cancer cells can be injected into the body of a suspected sufferer where they will home in on the antigen on the cancer cells. They can be labelled with a radioactive isotope, so that when the patient is scanned later on with a gamma radiation scanner it will be possible to see where they have found most of the antigen. These pictures are rather difficult to interpret, because not only is there antigen on the tumour, it will also have been shed from the tumour cells into the circulating bloodstream, and so a substantial proportion of the radioactive antibody will also remain in the blood, confusing the picture. One solution being tried is to inject another radioactive isotope into the blood just before the picture is taken. If the signal from this second isotope is taken to represent the blood and is subtracted from the signal from the radioactively-labelled antibody, the resulting picture should give a much clearer indication of the whereabouts of the cancer, see page 42.

After a tumour has been removed surgically, or treated with radiation, there is always the possibility that it will regrow, or that a secondary tumour will develop somewhere else in the body, and a regular check of cancer-associated antigens in the blood can give early warning of a recurrence.

Bone marrow transplants

Bone marrow transplants are used in treating leukaemia and other forms of cancer and also for other blood disorders, like immune deficiencies. It is a much simpler process than it sounds, because it does not involve cutting open the bones. The marrow can be extracted through needles, normally from the breastbone and hips, and then it is fed through a drip into the recipient's bloodstream. It will find its own way to the bones. The marrow for transplanting can come from one of two sources: from a donor, as in other transplants, or it can be the patient's own marrow. A transplant of the patient's own marrow is often done as part of the treatment of cancer. When somebody undergoes radiation or chemotherapy the factor that limits the intensity of the treatment is usually the bone marrow, because its cells are more vulnerable to damage than any others in the body. So to allow more aggressive treatment a proportion of the patient's bone marrow is sometimes removed and stored while the treatment is given and then returned. The problem with this is that even if the cancer is not one that principally affects the bone marrow (like leukaemia, for instance), but is a cancer, say, of the breast or lung, there may well be a few cancer cells lurking in the bone marrow and once it is returned these will grow. Using appropriate monoclonal antibodies as hooks it may well be possible to fish these dangerous cells out of the stored marrow before returning it.

If the reason for the transplant is that the patient's own bone marrow is diseased then the marrow for transplant will need to come from a donor, and if it is not perfectly matched he is in danger of a reaction called graft versus host disease (GVHD). As its name implies, this is a disease where the implanted bone marrow, which produces all the cells involved in the immune system, mounts an attack on the recipient of the transplant. The cells responsible for this attack are the T-lymphocytes, and if all the mature T-lymphocytes are removed from the donated marrow (and there is an MCA that can distinguish mature T-cells from others) then there is less risk that GVHD will develop.

In either case the antibodies will attach themselves to the unwanted cells, but there is still the problem of separating them out. A variety of

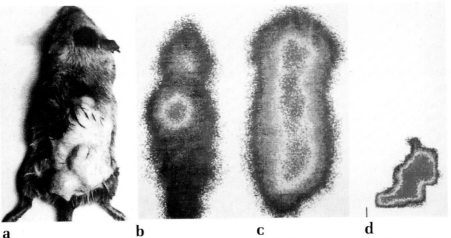

a   b   c   d

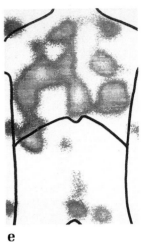

e

Locating a tumour using radioactively marked monoclonal antibodies: (a) A mouse has a tumour on its back; (b) first radioactive injection (which stays in the blood) shows how the blood is distributed about the mouse's body; (c) radioactively labelled antibody injection shows distribution of antigen in tumour and blood; (d) Image shows the tumour after the activity due to the antibody in blood has been subtracted; (e) using the same principle the spread of a cancer is revealed in the lungs and liver of a human patient, see page 41.

methods of doing the job have been tried, but one ingenious idea involves the use of magnets. The antibodies are attached firmly to tiny metal spheres before they are added to the bone marrow. Then the mixture is thoroughly stirred for some time to allow the antibodies to seek out all the target cells. After that the bone marrow is passed through a magnetic field which pulls out all the metal particles complete with their attached antibodies and cells. The same effect can be achieved by using the antibody to trigger a chemical attack to kill the cells, or by attaching the antibodies to a solid surface or the surface of some kind of filter.

A bullet with cancer's name on it?

The ultimate in cancer treatments, a monoclonal antibody targeted exclusively to a cancer and attached to a powerful poison, sounds too good to be true. At the moment it is not true, but it could be on its way. The earliest experiments in making these latest versions of the magic bullet have used two extremely powerful poisons: ricin, a product of the castor oil bean; and diphtheria toxin, the weapon used by the diphtheria microbe to kills its victim. The first difficulty facing the researchers who have been attempting to build these magic bullets was that even if the antibody would only react with cancer cells, it had very little chance of getting there, because the other part, the ricin or diphtheria molecule, reacted all too readily with normal cells: that is why it is such an effective poison.

This first stumbling block was overcome surprisingly easily. Both the ricin and the diphtheria toxin molecule turned out to be in two parts: one, the A part, carries the poisonous quality; the other, the B chain, the ability to attach itself to cells. So by splitting the molecule in two and using only the A chains, the poison could be prevented from killing the normal healthy cells.

The immunotoxins, as these combined molecules are called, could now find their way to tumour cells very well, but the trouble was that they were much less poisonous than they should have been. This, it turned out, was because the B chain of the poison molecule carried not only the ability to attach the molecule to the cell, but also the ability to move inside the cell where it could play its lethal role. The antibody, it seemed, did not have this ability, so the poison was often remaining on the outside of the cell and having little or no effect.

The researchers did not let this little setback stop them. The part of the poison molecule that had this ability to penetrate cells must be found, and put back. One way to do this would be to go back to the whole poison molecule and try to cut out not the whole of the B chain, but only the particular section that linked it to the normal cells. To date no one has succeeded in doing this – although the researchers are still trying. However, there is now another way of approaching a task like this. The diphtheria bacterium contains in its genes a sequence that controls the making of the toxin. If that genetic blueprint could be modified, cutting out only the sequence that fixes the poison to normal cells, then the remaining gene could be put back into a bacterium and grown, and the bacterium would produce a suitably modified poison. This has now been done, which gives another impetus to the search for specific cancer antibodies.

Work with monoclonal antibodies is only just beginning, and it is quite possible that some of the present ideas for their use in medicine will turn out to be unworkable, although it is equally likely that they will prove useful in ways that cannot yet be imagined. But their most

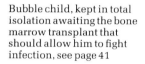

Bubble child, kept in total isolation awaiting the bone marrow transplant that should allow him to fight infection, see page 41

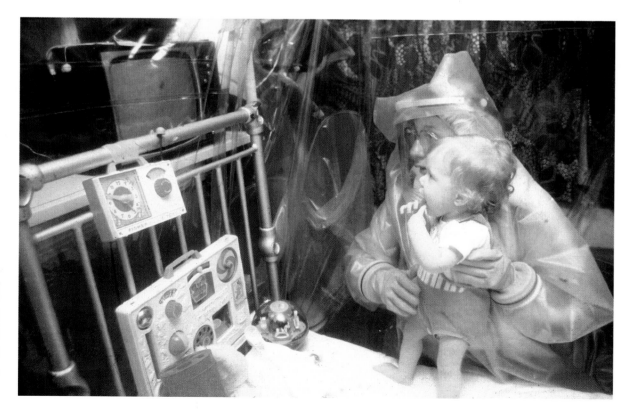

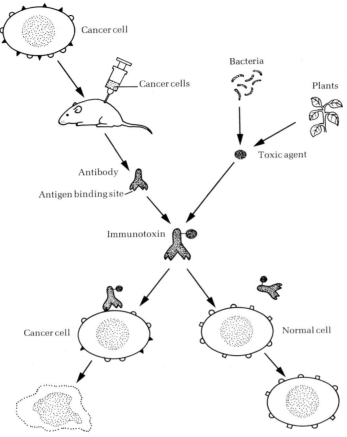

Cancer cell

Cancer cells

Bacteria

Plants

Toxic agent

Antibody

Antigen binding site

Immunotoxin

Cancer cell

Normal cell

How to make a magic bullet, or immunotoxin, see page 42.

valuable contribution could well turn out to be not in any particular application in diagnosis or cure, but in the field of basic research. MCAs should provide a powerful tool for scientists studying the immune system. By separating out all the components of the cells and chemical signals involved in the immune response, they may at last be able to understand precisely what is going on in the diseases where the immune system becomes over-zealous, the auto-immune diseases; or turned down or switched off, as in AIDS, the frightening condition that has hit the headlines in the past few years.

'Own goals': the auto-immune diseases

An auto-immune disease is one in which the immune system begins to treat part of its own body's tissue as an invader. It is only quite recently that a number of common and extremely serious diseases have been identified as belonging to this group, among them multiple sclerosis, the type of diabetes that attacks children, rheumatoid arthritis and all the related rheumatic diseases. It is believed that the disease process starts with an infection of some kind, although in most cases it is not known what infectious organism is responsible. In rheumatoid arthritis the latest candidate is a member of a group called parvoviruses, and its discoverers are confident enough to have called it RA1; it has been found in the joints of sufferers from the disease in both Britain and the United States. In diabetes it is thought that it may possibly be the Coxsackie virus, which has a tendency to go to the organ involved in diabetes, the pancreas. In other diseases the organism is still completely unknown, and indeed it is not certain that the process necessarily starts with an infection.

One possible picture of how an auto-immune disease might develop assumes that when the infectious organism invades the body it damages a particular group of cells: in the joints in rheumatoid arthritis, the nerves in multiple sclerosis, or the pancreas in diabetes. This damage is enough to change the cells so much that they will no longer be recognizable as self, and thereafter the immune system is continuously armed to fight them. Why the damage done by these viruses should lead to an auto-immune disease in some people and not in others who are also infected is not known, but it seems likely to be connected in some way with the HLA system (see page 00). This is because people with a particular mix of HLA system antigens are much more likely to develop this type of disease, although the mix for each disease appears to be different, and any of the diseases can happen to people who do not have the characteristic antigens. Nevertheless, it is thought that the connection may be that the initial infection and the HLA antigens together produce a structure which the immune system can no longer recognize, and it and all other cells like it become targets. There are all kinds of questions still to be answered, such as whether it is the recognition or the signalling that goes wrong, whether it is the switching on of the system or the failure to switch off that is at fault, and it is these questions that monoclonal antibodies might well help to answer.

Even without full details there are strategies for treatment if not cure of these problems. If childhood-onset diabetes really is an auto-immune disease, and it can be definitely established which virus or viruses are responsible, then it may be possible to vaccinate the most vulnerable children, possibly even using an engineered multiple vaccine if more than one organism is involved. In both multiple sclerosis and diabetes trials are taking place of the effect of using drugs that suppress the immune system. Another strategy being worked on for the future involves growing monoclonal antibodies to the immune cells which the body is producing to attack itself. These anti-antibodies could inactivate only the particular immune cells that the body has programmed to attack itself, leaving the rest of the system intact to protect it against other types of disease.

If the auto-immune disease is one where much of the damage is being caused not by armed T-cells but by B-cells making anti-self antibody, then there is another possible treatment: filtering out the antibodies from the blood. Antigens can be stuck on to a filter to hook out antibodies as the blood is passed through, but there is a problem – the antigen will not only attract the antibody, it will also attract B- and T-lymphocytes and provoke even more antibodies and higher immune activity, making the situation worse. A group in West Germany have solved that problem by developing a special filter containing a membrane which has pores large enough to allow the antibodies through to attach themselves to the antigens coating the tube wall, but too small to allow the much larger lymphocytes to make contact. Although the original problem would still exist and the system would make more antibody, this filter should considerably reduce the amount of damage done by the disease.

AIDS

The first case in the epidemic of acquired immune deficiency syndrome (AIDS) in the United States is thought to have been in 1978, although it was not until the summer of 1981 that people began to realize there was a serious problem. The disease broke out in the homosexual communities of San Francisco and New York. In the eyes of some people it was seen as a punishment from God (rather as diseases like syphilis had been, according to the thinking of earlier centuries) and even the more down-to-earth doctors dealing with the early cases of the disease thought it probably had something to do with the homosexual life style – perhaps a result of drug abuse or promiscuity, or perhaps both.

AIDS is not so much a disease as a condition in which a selection of peculiar diseases can develop. The most common is Kaposi's sarcoma, a cancer of the skin and mucous membranes, which before AIDS was only met in a mild form in some elderly people, but was virtually unknown in the virulent form in which it attacks the young AIDS victims. There is also a type of pneumonia, caused by an organism which is common but normally harmless, and a variety of infections which until AIDS were only known to attack animals. What sufferers from all these diseases have in common is that their immune system breaks down; the balance is upset between two sets of T-lymphocytes, the T-helper cells which activate the whole immune reaction, and the T-suppressor cells which switch it off. In healthy people there are twice as many helpers as suppressors, in AIDS the balance is the other way round.

The idea that this breakdown was due in some way to the homosexual way of life was upset when the disease began to appear in a few isolated people who had no connection at all with homosexuals. Among them were a number of sufferers from haemophilia, and it soon became clear that the one thing this group had in common was that they had all had transfusions of blood, or in the case of the haemophiliacs of the factor that is needed for the blood to clot. This suggested that the cause of the disease was an infection, and one that could be passed in the blood. It was very difficult to isolate the responsible organism, because the failure of the patients' immune systems meant that their bodies were

Particles of HTLV III, the
virus associated with AIDS

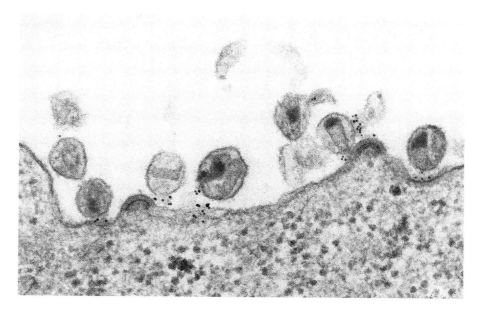

riddled with all kinds of infections. However, teams in France and the United States have now isolated organisms which they are fairly sure are responsible. The two teams have given their organisms different names – in France it is LAV and in America HTLV III – but they are almost certainly versions of the same organism.

These viruses may turn out to be only part of the explanation of AIDS, because they have not yet been found in all sufferers from the condition, and it seems certain that not everyone infected with the organism(s) gets the disease. Nevertheless, biotechnology companies in the United States are already working on vaccines, and one company suggested it would have a vaccine ready to begin tests by midsummer 1985. However that looks very optimistic now, because it seems likely that the AIDS virus may be very variable (rather like the flu virus).

Meanwhile doctors have been working on possible ways of treating the unfortunates who have already been infected, and they have concentrated particularly on people who show signs of the T-cell imbalance but do not yet have any of the potentially fatal conditions that often follow. Since the deficiency is in the immune system they started treating the patients with chemicals which are produced by the body as part of the immune reaction: interferon and interleukin-2. They had high hopes particularly of interleukin-2, because that is the chemical the body uses to instruct T-cells to grow. (It is sometimes known as T-cell growth factor.) But so far the best results appear to come from another treatment, an anti-viral drug, which does seem to be able to restore the balance in the T-cells. The improvement seems to continue after the treatment stops, and the doctor who has been using the drug thinks it is in some way stimulating the bone marrow to make new, healthy T-cells. Whether this can be called a cure, and whether it will help those who are already affected by the dreadful second stage of the disease, are both questions that have not yet been answered.

Interferon and lymphokines

Interferon has see-sawed between being a miracle drug that could cure cancer and infectious disease, and being useless – and back again, more than once in the almost 30 years since it was discovered. It is the body's own antiviral, but is unusual in that it is not only produced by the specialist cells of the immune system, but also by ordinary structural cells.

When a virus enters a cell it begins to reproduce and continues making copies of itself until the cell is destroyed and its contents released. At that moment a tiny amount of interferon is released by the dying cell, and this signals to all the neighbouring cells telling them to arm against invaders. How the message is then passed from cell to cell is not known, but the thing that makes interferon particularly interesting to its supporters is that, unlike the products of the specialist cells, interferon has the ability to arm cells against a large range of invaders, not only the one that started the reaction. Since it also affects the growth of cancer cells it has great theoretical possibilities.

The reason why there is still so much uncertainty about its real value is that until very recently it was impossible to produce enough interferon to do the necessary research. Animal interferon does not work in humans, so it had to be extracted from human cells, where it is produced in minute quantities. But many more facts have begun to appear now that the gene for the chemical has been stitched into bacteria and it is being made in large quantities.

It is proving to be much more complicated than it at first seemed. There are at least three different types in humans, and their effects are very mixed. Small and large doses can produce opposite reactions, and so can similar doses given at different times. Another problem is that the chemical seems to have worse side effects than the researchers hoped, ranging from flu-like symptoms to much more severe reactions, and even coma. In a rare cancer called hairy-cell leukaemia interferon appears to be very effective, but in other cancers its effects are still uncertain. It has some effect in a number of viral infections, and shows signs of being able to prevent, if not to cure, the common cold – no mean achievement considering how many other methods have failed.

Interferon is just one of the immune signalling chemicals, the lymphokines, that are now being mass-produced by biotechnology, and others may prove to be of more value. Among them are chemicals the body uses to call up phagocytes, inhibit the growth of cancer cells, and instruct lymphocytes to grow, and there will be more. A whole new road is opening up and in the next few years we should begin to know whether it leads somewhere exciting.

CHAPTER THREE
How It Hurts

The ability to feel pain is a vital one. Sufferers from diseases like leprosy who have ceased to feel pain do enormous damage to hands, feet and other parts simply because they no longer notice the injuries like burns and blisters that make most of us stop what we are doing because it hurts. We should therefore be grateful that we have the pain early-warning system; but unfortunately when we have received and taken note of the warning we have only very imperfect ways of switching the alarm off. This would not matter so much if pain only occurred as a result of an injury, and went away as soon as the wound was healed. However, there are several types of severe pain, like that of arthritis or cancer, which can last for a very long time, and the treatment of that chronic pain is extremely difficult.

Even the severest short term pain is no longer a problem. Everyone is afraid when facing surgery, but it is no longer fear of feeling pain during the operation itself. People tell horror stories of patients who could hear all the surgeons were saying while the operation was going on. Probably at least half of them are apocryphal, but even if they were all true it would not necessarily matter very much, because the ability to feel pain is one of the very first faculties to go under a general anaesthetic. We hold on to hearing, sight, even touch, much more tenaciously. And not everybody chooses to be unconscious during an operation. Nowadays even quite major surgery is done under only a local anaesthetic and, if he so chooses, a hernia patient can watch in the mirror above the table as the surgeon neatly darns the weak patch in his abdominal wall. Local

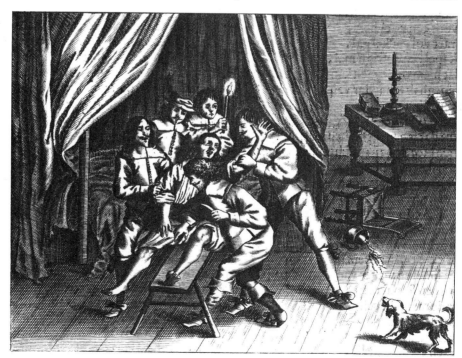

Surgery in pre-anaesthetic days. Amputations were often performed with nothing more than alcohol to reduce the pain

anaesthetics on this scale, as well as other advances in pain control, have developed following improvements in our understanding of how pain works.

The classic picture of how we experience pain was quite simple. A foot or hand touches the fire, the message goes to the brain, and it is experienced as pain. So far as it goes, that is quite correct, except that the process is, of course, much more complicated. Pain signals start from the nerves, which are distributed all over the body. They are not evenly spaced, far from it, but there is nowhere on the normal human anatomy that you can prick with a pin without eliciting a protest. Normally it is when the ends of nerves are stimulated that we feel pain, and as babies we learn to distinguish between signals from different nerves. We also have nerves which pick up signals inside the body. Although we are unable to feel the sensation of our intestines working or our hearts beating, we can feel some pain originating inside us. One particular stimulus, the stretching of a vessel or duct which is blocked, sends an extremely powerful signal to the brain. Another pain that can give a useful warning is that which comes from a muscle deprived of adequate oxygen supplies. Angina, the pain from the heart muscle, is probably the most severe.

There are, however, many peculiar types of pain, and questions about them have puzzled people for a long time. We all know how violent the pain can be from stepping on a drawing pin or touching a piece of hot metal. What must be a minor stimulus involving just a few nerves can make us feel quite sick with pain. But we have also heard stories of soldiers in battle carrying on with ghastly wounds, or football players in the heat of their sort of battle continuing with broken limbs. If the pinprick stimulus was simply multiplied by the number of nerves involved, the pain from injuries of this sort would be overwhelming. Yet soldiers on the Anzio beaches in the Second World War are reported as saying that they did not feel their wounds.

There are other things that are even more difficult to explain if pain is the simple result of a nerve ending being damaged and sending a message to the brain signalling distress. There are peculiar things like phantom limb pain, where an amputated limb continues to hurt long after the stump has healed. There are strange diseases where a succession of harmless sensations like moderate heat can be added together in some way to give a feeling like burning. An attack of shingles can leave in its wake a dreadful condition where a tiny stimulus, no more than blowing on the skin perhaps, can cause agonizing pain. And there are other, even stranger types of pain that can be triggered by a gentle touch but not by stabbing with a pin.

To fit all these peculiarities into a theory of how pain works has proved very difficult, and the precise mechanism by which some of them arise is still a long way from being understood. But in the 1960s a Canadian psychologist called Ronald Melzack and a British anatomist,

Descartes believed that pain signals from the limbs travelled up hollow tubes (the nerves) directly to the brain

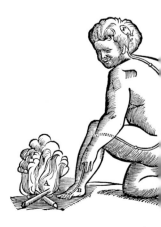

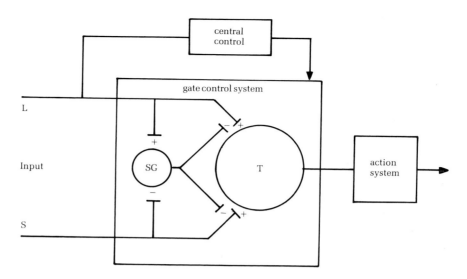

The Gate Control System. Both large and small fibres (L and S) send pain signals to the transmitter (T) which passes them on to the brain. But in the substantia gelatinosa (SG) is a 'gate' mechanism that can reduce the flow of pain signals. This mechanism is stimulated into action by signals from the large fibres

Patrick Wall, suggested a system which is accepted by the majority of workers in the field. What is more, it has led to developments in the way that pain is treated. It is called the Gate Theory of Pain, and it works like this.

Before a message can get from the site of an injury to the brain, where it can be experienced as pain, it has to go through a gate. How severe the pain feels will depend on how wide open the gate is. That depends on a number of factors. First, the nerve fibres that carry the pain signals from the skin come in two varieties, large and small. They both carry pain signals, but both also have an effect on the gate. Whereas the small fibres tend to push the gate open, the large fibres tend to push it shut. In addition it seems that stimulation of the large fibres sends a warning direct to some kind of higher control system which in turn will act to shut the gate. At the same time the brain itself is sending down signals which also affect the condition of the gate.

Melzack and Wall have not yet produced a full picture of how the gate system actually modifies the signal from the nerves, but they think it happens just as the signal enters the spinal cord, in a part called the substantia gelatinosa. It is then passed to a transmission cell which sends it up to the brain. So the part of the brain where pain is actually 'felt' receives only this fully processed pattern of impulses. And it is this pattern that determines whether the signals are felt as pain, and if so how bad it is.

Given that explanation of how the system works, how does it help with the task of treating unwanted pain?

Drugs

Most of the drugs we have available for dealing with pain today are very similar to the ones that have been around for centuries. One that has enjoyed a long and honourable career is aspirin.

There are suggestions that it may first have been used, in its natural state, by Hippocrates, the 'Father of Medicine', in 400 BC. It was an English clergyman called Edward Stone who made the first written report that we know of on the virtues of the extract of the willow tree that later came to be known as aspirin. His report went to The Royal Society in 1763. The story goes that he was looking for a treatment for intermittent fevers. Since they tended to occur in damp areas it was reasonable for a man of the cloth to assume that the good Lord would provide a cure among the plants growing in watery areas. The willow grows alongside streams, and so . . .

Chemists isolated the active principle, which they named salicin after salix, the willow. They worked on the molecule to get rid of some of its irritant properties, and they learned to synthesize their best version, acetylsalicilic acid, which we now know as aspirin. Although we have been taking aspirin tablets by the million for nearly a hundred years its mode of action was completely unknown until recently. It was not even known whether it acted locally at the site of the pain or in the brain itself.

In the late 1960s and early 1970s Dr John Vane of the Royal College of Surgeons in London made a discovery which showed how it worked at the site of the injury. The most common use for aspirin is probably for headache, and after that toothache. Much stronger aspirin is given to sufferers from arthritis and other pain associated with inflammation, which is the body's response to any damage to its tissues. Inflammation affects the local blood vessels, causing redness, but it also makes the local nerve endings much more sensitive; hence the pain. But the body does not produce this response as a direct result of injury. There is an intermediary. When the cell wall is damaged it releases a chemical which stimulates the production of a chemical messenger called a prostaglandin. It is the prostaglandin that in its turn triggers the in-flammation response, and aspirin works by preventing, or at least inhibiting, the production of prostaglandin. Since prostaglandin is also involved in triggering the complicated mechanism involved in headache, it now seems we have at least part of the explanation.

To treat the severest type of pain, like the pain of terminal cancer, calls for something stronger than aspirin. The most effective drugs we know for dealing with that level of pain without rendering the sufferer unconscious are still the ones derived from the opium poppy, heroin and morphine. Although they, too, have been in use for many centuries, again it is only in the last 20 years that their action has been understood; and it is totally different from the aspirin type. It seems that the opiates work in the gate itself, and in the brain. The shape of the morphine or heroin molecule is such that it can lock on to specific receptors inside the spinal cord and brain, and prevent the passing on of pain signals.

This was a very surprising finding. What possible reason could there be for the presence in the human central nervous system of receptors specifically designed to fit molecules from the poppy? The answer, of course, is that the poppy is an intruder. The receptors are designed to be triggered by chemicals made in the brain itself. They were found in the late 1970s and called endorphins (endogenous morphines) and en-kephalins. It seems certain now that these endorphins are part of the natural mechanism for closing the gate. The fact that the shape of the molecule in the poppy allows it to perform the same function is pure accident, although the Revd Edward Stone might see it as part of a Grand Design.

As everyone knows, morphine and heroin have their drawbacks. The main one is that as well as relieving pain they also cause euphoria and strange psychedelic effects. Some people find these effects pleasant, others find them very unpleasant. Another problem is that all the opiates are highly addictive.

In the eighteenth and nineteenth centuries every well-equipped household kept laudanum, an opiate, along with the smelling salts; there was even a special version for children. Earlier this century there was a reaction against the opiates. Doctors began to worry about addiction, and it was believed that the effect of the drugs would diminish so that larger and larger doses would be needed to cope with the same level of pain. It is difficult to see that either of these was a good reason for refusing a drug to a dying person, and now the opiates are back in favour. The hospice movement has reminded doctors that the overwhelming need of the dying is to be free of pain. What is more, a careful study of the drugs in use in the treatment of terminal pain has shown that their pain-killing effect does not diminish; stronger doses are only needed if the pain becomes greater.

After the discovery of the naturally occurring opiates, the endorphins and enkephalins, there was hope that the pharmaceutical industry might be able to sidestep any traces of this conflict that remain. Some of the enkephalins are really quite small molecules which could be easily synthesized. It was hoped that by using manufactured copies of these it might be possible to produce the relief of pain without any of the other effects, and therefore without any danger of addiction. But unfortunately it did not work. Trials so far have shown that the man-made copies of natural opiates engender all the same effects as the products of the poppy, including the undesirable ones. So the perfect opiate, as well as the perfect anti-inflammatory drug still remains elusive.

Surgery

There are some types of pain that resist all attempts to treat them adequately with drugs. These are the types that result from damage to nerves which either never heal or regrow in such a way that they send out continuous pain signals. Phantom limb pain and the pain following shingles are both problems of this sort, and until recently, once drugs had failed, the only way of treating them was by breaking the pathway of the nerves in some way. This can be done by cutting, or more often by destroying the fibres chemically, or by burning or freezing. Sometimes these procedures are very effective, but they can make the situation worse, and following the gate theory we can understand why. If the pain originates from a small area and the nerves are destroyed before they reach the spinal cord, then the ill effects may follow from an upset of the balance between small and large fibres. If the pain is spread over a large area then the interruption can be made as the nerves enter the spinal cord or even in the cord itself. But then the body's own moderating influences, like the endorphins and enkephalins, may be interfered with. So although interruption of the fibres can be very successful, it is perfectly possible for surgery to make matters worse.

Although attempts at permanent blocking of nerve signals in the spinal cord have not always been successful, temporary blocking with a local anaesthetic has been in use for 20 years in childbirth and to help post-operative pain. More recently it has become increasingly common as the only anaesthetic – apart from a mild sedative – for quite major surgery. It is called epidural anaesthesia, because the anaesthetic is put into the epidural space. The spinal cord itself is enclosed in a tough tube called the dura which is filled with cerebro-spinal fluid. Between that and the bones of the spine, the vertebrae, is a space, the epidural space. The anaesthetist puts a needle into that space at the same level as the nerves he wants to block. The nerves have to pass through that space to get into the spinal cord, so he bathes them in local anaesthetic, which blocks the passage of any signals. This temporary block seems to have none of the uncertainty attached to permanent damage. It appears always to produce the desired effect. The local anaesthetic only lasts for a few hours, although if the needle is left in place it can be kept topped up. But the topping up can go on for only a few days. After that the

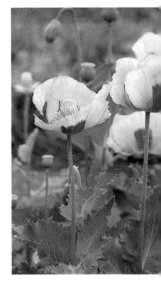

ABOVE Papaver Sominiferum. The opium poppy, source of one of the oldest drugs

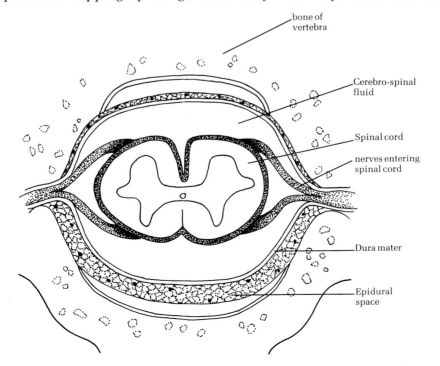

bone of vertebra

Cerebro-spinal fluid

Spinal cord

nerves entering spinal cord

Dura mater

Epidural space

LEFT Cross section of the spinal column showing the epidural space where drugs are injected to anaesthetise a part of the body for childbirth or surgery

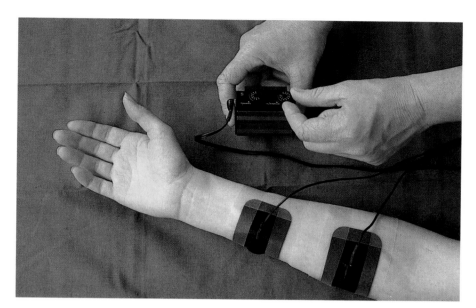

ABOVE TENS. The effect of
Transcutaneous Electrical
Nerve Stimulation in
controlling pain in the
forearms is assessed by a
hospital physiotherapist
RIGHT Acupuncture points
and meridians as detailed in
a Chinese textbook

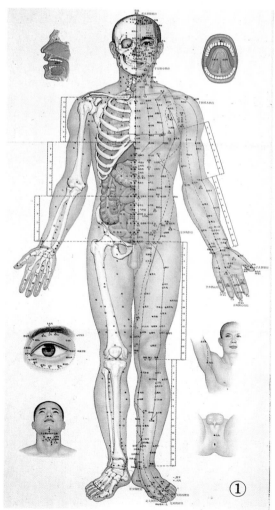

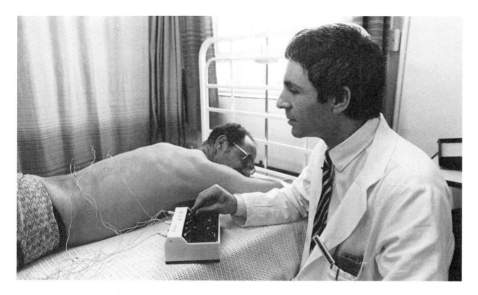

Electro-acupuncture in use
at St Bartholomew's
Hospital, London

anaesthetic agent begins to damage the nerves, risking the same ill effects as can result from deliberate destruction; and in any case it would not be an ideal permanent treatment, because this sort of block affects all types of feeling, not only pain.

Any attempt to interrupt the nerves in this way, whether temporarily or permanently, must involve some risk. The introduction of the gate control theory has suggested that there might be some rationale for a very long-established way of dealing with pain, and has led to its modern refinement.

Kiss it better
Depending on who is doing the kissing, the effect of this may be a more general distraction. But applying a local stimulus, like scratching or a good rub, is our instinctive way of dealing with an itch or a pain. What we are probably trying to do is stimulate the large fibres in order to close the gate. Certain types of stimulus quite definitely do excite the large (moderating) fibres more than the small (intensifying) ones. Electrical stimulation is one of them, since current flows more easily through the large fibres. Patrick Wall, one of the founding fathers of the gate control theory, therefore decided to try stimulating large fibres, both on the skin and with electrodes in the spinal cord. The results were good enough for the electrical stimulator to have become the first choice in the treatment of some types of pain.

One injury is seen all too often in young motorcyclists. Travelling at speed, they collide with a fixed object or a moving vehicle and are thrown over the handlebars of their machine. The natural instinct is to hold on, with at least one hand. The result is that the arm is wrenched severely and the nerves are torn, stretched, even pulled out of their connection in the cord. Although attempts are made as far as possible to restore some use to the arm, one of the worst problems is often pain from the damaged nerves, which goes on and on; and one of the best ways of dealing with this has proved to be electrical stimulation from electrodes placed on the skin. Transdermal electrical nerve stimulation, as it is called, is now used for many types of pain, from pulled muscles in athletes to the severe pain suffered by the accident victims.

Another effect of the gate theory, and of the discovery of the body's home-made analgesics, the endorphins, has been to provide a possible explanation, and therefore orthodox medical respectability, for techniques like hypnosis and acupuncture, as well as for psychological approaches.

Acupuncture

Traditional Chinese acupuncture involves inserting needles, now usually of stainless steel, but sometimes gold, through the skin to a depth of about 25 mm (1 in), and then twisting them round and round. Sometimes a substance called moxa is attached to the needle and ignited. This is called moxibustion and is designed to enhance the effect of the acupuncture. The needles must be inserted at very specific points depending on which part of the body is ailing, but the acupuncture point for a given part is normally some distance from it, and the two are connected by a meridian. Unlike nerves or blood vessels there is no recognizable anatomical evidence of the meridians in the body, and the whole procedure is part of an elaborate and mystical theory. This may be why it has been rejected for so long in the West. But acupuncture unquestionably has an effect, at least in the relief of pain; and it is something more than simple suggestion since it works in animals.

It is now known that at least part of the effect of acupuncture is in stimulating the production of endorphins, because an increase in endorphins has been found in the cerebro-spinal fluid of patients given acupuncture for the relief of pain. What is more, a drug that prevents the action of endorphins also blocks the effects of acupuncture. This discovery, together with the result of a number of controlled trials of acupuncture for relief of pain, have won the needles a much more general acceptance in Britain, for example, so that now acupuncture is available on the National Health Service, from GPs and from hospitals. We still have no explanation of the nature of the meridians, and many people who use acupuncture do not think that success depends on observing them, or on using only the points shown on the charts — although some points certainly are more effective than others.

Electrical stimulation and acupuncture are obviously treatments which, when they work, are much less risky than surgical or chemical destruction of nerves, and they would seem to be preferable to dependence on drugs. There might, however, be an even better method, if only we knew how to harness it. If soldiers and footballers can ignore broken limbs, then the body must be capable of producing its own very powerful analgesia. Psychology, lessons in relaxation, harnessing the placebo effect: a combination of these could turn out to be the best solution of all in reducing the destructive effects of long-term severe pain.

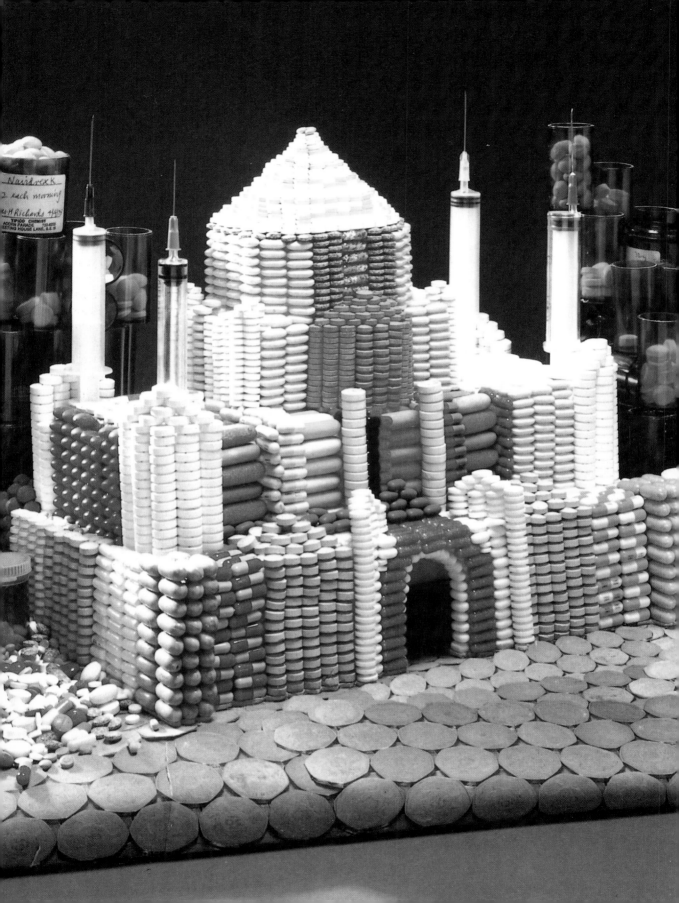

Chemical Solutions

OPPOSITE The building blocks of the drug industry

The modern drug industry was born out of the dyestuffs industry at the end of the nineteenth century, with the hunt for chemicals to fight the newly discovered organisms that cause infectious disease. Chemists decided to try an alternative to the system which had produced most of the drugs available up to that time: hunting through nature as the Revd Stone had done to find drugs to reduce symptoms. The new 'chemo-therapy' would create its own chemical magic bullets, and these magic bullets would cure the disease itself.

Paul Ehrlich (1854–1915), the German bacteriologist and immunologist, was the man who founded this line of research. He worked in a laboratory dealing with infectious disease and his interest in chemicals was born out of his experiments with dyes. A variety of dyes were used to stain the bacteria to make them easier to see under the microscope. Ehrlich had observed how the various organisms seemed to have a particular affinity for different dyes. If an organism would take up a chemical that was not taken up by the cells of the host, then it should be possible to produce a magic bullet, a chemical that would go into a bacterium and kill it, but leave the human or animal host undamaged.

The first major disease to succumb to Ehrlich's approach was syphilis. At that time syphilis was an appalling scourge, causing one in ten deaths in some parts of Europe. In its later stages it produced terrible symptoms ranging from madness and paralysis to rotting ulcers. Ehrlich started work on the microbe that was the cause of syphilis with a chemical related to arsenic. He had heard reports that this chemical had some effect on similar micro-organisms. First Ehrlich tried the chemical itself, then his laboratory began making every modification he could think of to the molecule. It was the six hundred and sixth derivative that finally proved to have the desired effect. It killed the organisms, leaving the infected animals (they were rabbits) unharmed.

BELOW LEFT The spirochaete which causes syphilis, the first infectious disease to be treated successfully with a tailor-made drug
BELOW RIGHT Round a patch of pencillium mould is a clear area where penicillin from the mould has prevented the growth of bacteria

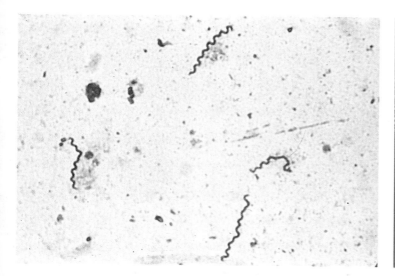

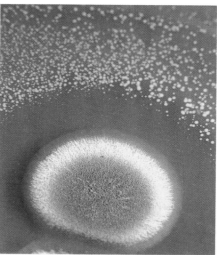

Ehrlich called his magic bullet Salvarsan and testing began. To a society like ours that agonizes over the morality of allowing prisoners or medical students to take part in drug research (can their participation ever be truly voluntary?), reports of the testing of Salvarsan are quite incredible. Any of the local prostitutes suffering from the disease were compulsorily treated with Salvarsan, by force if necessary, and despite the fact that unskilful injections could cause serious damage to tissue. There were some amputations of limbs damaged by careless injections, and deaths were laid at the door of Salvarsan, although the link was never proved. Nevertheless, it did cure large numbers of people who without it would have progressed to an early and extremely unpleasant death.

Although Salvarsan was never the magic bullet Ehrlich hoped, for some years the only progress in treatment of bacterial disease came from other chemical companies following Ehrlich's technique using dyes. But the real 'breakthrough' in antibacterial discovery came from an approach that looks more like the old system: looking for remedies in nature.

The discovery of penicillin is probably the best publicized 'accident' in the history of science. But contamination of bacterial samples by moulds happened every day, and the important thing was that this particular case was reported by the British bacteriologist Alexander Fleming because he was at that time looking for natural 'antiseptics', although in plant and animal tissue rather than moulds. It created very little excitement at the time of its discovery (1928), because it was well

BELOW LEFT Alexander Fleming – the first man to take an interest in the ability of penicillium mould to kill bacteria
BELOW RIGHT Howard Florey, the leader of the team that turned penicillin into a life-saving drug

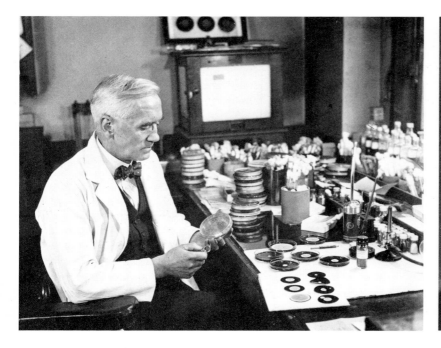
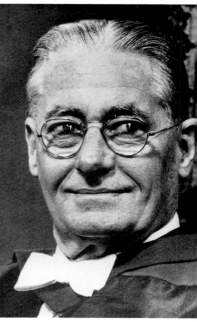

known that moulds could inhibit the growth of bacteria. Fleming's mould was, however, a particularly effective one, and he was convinced that it was useful, if not to medicine, then certainly to bacteriologists. So he publicized it, and made sure it survived by sending cultures all over the country; but whereas penicillin was undoubtedly Fleming's discovery, penicillin the drug that saved countless lives and led to a generation of antibiotics, resulted from the work of Howard Florey and his team at Oxford. Receiving very little encouragement from anyone (including Fleming), in a heroic effort, using milk churns and bedpans to contain their cultures and purify their solutions (it was wartime and proper equipment was unobtainable), they showed that this substance was not just another antiseptic. Since penicillin all major antibacterial medicines have taken a substance found in nature as their starting point.

At the moment there are no major bacterial diseases for which we have no effective antibiotic, yet no one regards the war as having been won. There were so few undesirable side effects from antibiotics that until about 15 years ago any that could be made cheaply enough were used with gay abandon. Intensively farmed animals were given blanket antibiotics to prevent the development of disease which could easily spread through the whole stock. Humans would nip off to the doctor for an antibiotic at the first snuffle, regardless of whether it was appropriate: and usually it was not.

The nasty shock came when diseases which had been easily treatable with antibiotics suddenly appeared to be able to persist. It seemed that resistant strains were developing. At first it was assumed that this was simply natural selection at work. People were taking antibiotics for a short time, but stopping as soon as their symptoms had vanished. This left the bacteria with least susceptibility to that particular antibiotic alive to fight another day. So antibiotic takers were urged that they must always finish any course of antibiotics.

Survival of the fittest was not, however, the full explanation of the newly resistant bacteria. Resistance was appearing in diseases that had been 100 per cent treatable before, and it soon began to look as if one bug was able to pass on its resistance to another. Nobody knew how this could be done. Bacteria normally reproduce by cell division, producing two carbon copies of the original bacterium. Although accidental changes to the genes can take place during cell division, it seemed impossible that this explained how the bacteria acquired drug resistance. Then researchers studying bacteria under the microscope found that occasionally two bacteria seemed to be joined together by a thin tube. It turned out that these tubes were used to transmit tiny rings of bacterial genetic information (they were called plasmids) from one bacterium to another. At first it was assumed that this transfer could only happen between two bacteria of the same strain, that it was a sort of sexual mating. But later it was found that there were some plasmids

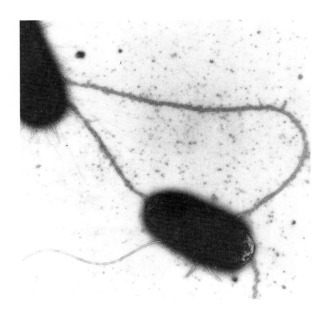

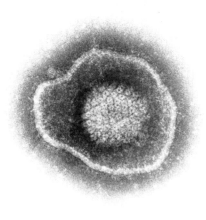

which contained a particular section of genetic material – they called it a 'jumping gene' – which allowed a plasmid to move between different strains of bacteria. It was with the help of these jumping genes that drug resistance was moving from one strain to another.

Drug resistance has appeared in a variety of diseases, ranging from widespread venereal infections at one end to malaria and leprosy at the other. Some of the most stubborn are the ones that lurk in hospitals to cause post-operative infections. Many hospitals have recently been seriously worried about a resistant strain of *Staphylococcus aureus*, a common cause of fatal septicaemia in the pre-penicillin days. So although antibiotics are a major success story, we now have to accept that we must restrict their use. What is more, the war against bacterial disease will never be completely won. The best we can hope for is to keep one step ahead of the microbes.

Viruses

The chemical war against viral disease has barely begun. Man has won a few battles, but so has the virus. The reason is that the hunt for medicines to treat infectious disease caused by bacteria was for many reasons a great deal easier. For a start, bacteria are easier to work with. They can be grown in a simple nutrient broth or on plates of jelly; and they are visible under the microscope.

Viruses are a different challenge altogether. To begin with most are so tiny that they were never seen at all until the invention of the electron microscope. Nor can they be grown in broth or on a gel plate. They are truly parasitic, and have to be given the living cells of some other organism to grow in. However, the greatest difference between bacteria and viruses, and the one that has given those searching for drugs to fight viruses most headaches, is the fact that viruses are simply lumps of genetic material wrapped up in a protein coat. They can do absolutely nothing for themselves, and their only function is to reproduce. Their

ABOVE LEFT Bacteria (*E. coli*) connected by two pili, the tubes through which genetic material passes from bacterium to bacterium
ABOVE RIGHT A herpes virus – a family that causes many kinds of disease, from shingles to cold sores

strategy is to move in on the cell of some host and commandeer the cell's chemical factory to enable them to make copies of their genetic material and of the protein units from which their coat is made.

Antibiotics are able to destroy bacteria because they interfere with the metabolism, the chemical activity through which the bacterium conducts its life. Since the bacterium is a separate entity it can be attacked and killed without necessarily damaging the cells of its host. But a virus that has taken over a cell in a human being is no longer a separate entity. It has incorporated itself completely into that cell, and so any antibiotic that damaged one would damage the other to an equal degree.

Until the 1960s the only thing a doctor could do for a sufferer from a viral disease was to send him to bed until his own defence mechanism, the immune system, had defeated the virus. A few drugs were developed that had some action against viruses, but they tended to attack many of the normal cells as well as the virus-infected ones, and unless the viral infection was extremely serious the cure was liable to be worse than the disease. In the 1970s a few more drugs were developed that had some effect against viruses, either by making it more difficult for them to get inside the cells of their potential victim, or by directly intensifying the action of the victim's immune system.

At the end of the 1970s came the beginning of a new type of antiviral. This type of drug should be as able to distinguish between normal cells and those invaded by viruses as the antibiotics were able to distinguish bacterial from host cells. The first, a drug that had a specific action against smallpox, was developed only months before smallpox itself was wiped out by other means. The second, launched at the end of 1979, was an extremely ingenious piece of work.

Acyclovir

Acyclovir, or 9-(2-Hydroxyethoxymethyl)guanine, to give it its full name, was designed to attack members of the herpes family of viruses. These cause a large variety of diseases, including cold sores, chicken-pox, shingles, and an extremely damaging type of eye disease, and they are even suspected of being the initial cause of some cancers. Herpes viruses are peculiar in that when a person is infected, he or she suffers from the typical 'weepy' sores, but after a while the immune system gains the upper hand, and they disappear. The virus, however, is not totally defeated. It retreats to the nerve cells where it remains quiet until its host is overtired, or stressed, or weakened in some other way, when the virus emerges and causes the sores again.

Acyclovir appears to be able to confine its attack very accurately to the cells that have been invaded by these viruses, and it singles them out by three different mechanisms. The first is that it finds it easier to get through the outer membrane of infected cells than normal ones. Then having entered a cell, it is only able to act if it finds signs that the virus has been at work. When a virus enters a cell it forces the cell to stop its normal activity and begin to make the virus's own versions of a number of important chemicals that will help in the manufacture of new protein and DNA to build new viruses. One of these chemicals is a particular form of an enzyme called thymidine kinase. Because this is made only on instructions from the virus it will be present only in cells invaded by the virus and not in normal ones. This is a vital difference, because the drug only becomes active in the presence of this viral enzyme. The enzyme changes the chemical form of the drug in such a way that it is 'armed' to interfere with the production of DNA. This is where the third level of the ability of the virus to single out the enemy comes in, because the drug appears to be between 10 and 30 times as efficient at interfering with the copying of viral types of DNA as it is in stopping the production of human DNA. This means that the virus is unable to do the one thing it lives for: to make copies of itself.

The drug does not kill the virus completely, so it can recur later; but it shortens the length of the time when the virus is active, and since that is when it is most infectious, the drug could reduce spread of the disease. Herpes comes in many different forms, and some are much more serious than others. Cold sores and genital herpes are distressing and unpleasant, but there is a form of herpes in the eye which causes ulcers, inflammation, and can result in blindness. Also some individuals are in particular danger from the virus. Anyone who has had a transplant must have his immune system put out of action so that he will not reject the transplanted organ. Since more than half of us have herpes virus particles hiding quietly somewhere in our nerves a transplant patient is likely to have them too, and the suppression of his immune system is the cue for the herpes to emerge and cause havoc. In these circumstances herpes can kill.

For these people a drug to treat the disease is absolutely vital, and that raises a problem. There are strains of herpes that are able to resist acyclovir – they do this by not making the right kind of thymidine kinase. The question is whether or not viruses, like bacteria, can acquire immunity. If they can, then widespread use of antiviral drugs might make them less able to help the few who have a vital need for them.

And so *ad infinitum*: bacteriophages

Bacteriophages, or phages, are viruses, but they are viruses that man is learning to look upon as potential allies rather than enemies, because the main targets for their attentions are bacteria, the sort of bacteria that can cause disease in man and animals. Phages treat bacteria in the same way as viruses treat human cells, invading them, and using the bacterial metabolism to create new phages. When enough of them have been made they burst open the bacterium. The idea of phage therapy is that someone infected with the kind of bacterium that causes an intestinal infection should swallow a dose of phages and leave them to get to work on the bacteria. It is not a new idea; it was first suggested very soon after

A bacterium (*E. coli*) under attack by an army of bacteriophages

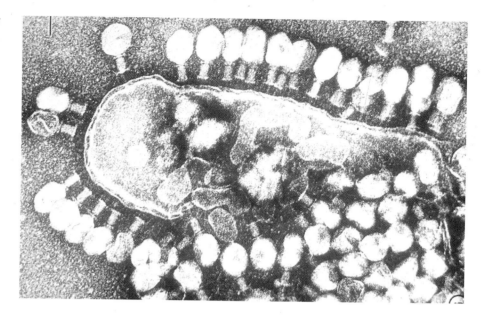

it was discovered that bacteria, too, had parasites preying on them. But early attempts to make use of phages did not work, and so it was abandoned. Then in 1983 microbiologists working with pigs, calves and sheep decided to give the idea another try, to see if they could find out why it had not worked. It may be simply that they are better at handling phages than their predecessors, but their results look much more promising. They have found that phages certainly do help to protect pigs against some intestinal infections; and at the moment there is no obvious reason why they should not be useful in treating intestinal disease in man too, like cholera and dysentery.

If phage treatment proves successful it may well have some advantages over antibiotic therapy. There do appear to be some resistant organisms but they are not very virulent and, of course, the phages could go on working even after bacteria have been excreted, which should help to prevent spread.

The developers of antibiotics and antivirals did, and do, have an advantage. The disease is caused by some kind of organism. Conquer the organism, and this should conquer the disease. But for many diseases there is no such enemy, and development of drugs calls for a different approach.

For much of the time the drug industry is trying to find better drugs to treat diseases whose cause is totally unknown. Until fairly recently most of them did this by refining, purifying and modifying substances taken from plants that had been prepared by herbalists for centuries. Nobody knows who first discovered that extract of foxglove leaves has a powerful effect on the heart. The fact was brought to the attention of

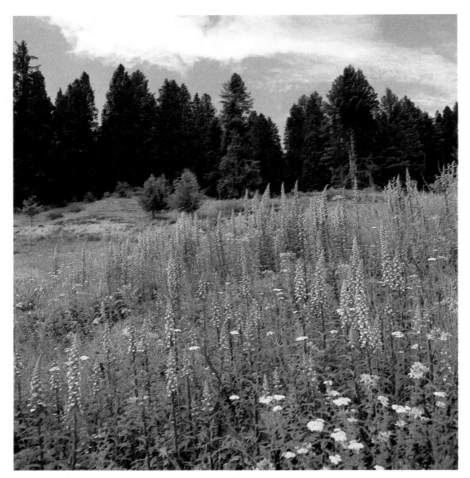

A field full of *Digitalis lanata*, the foxglove from which the drug digitalis or digoxin is produced

scientists and doctors at the end of the eighteenth century, and since then drug companies have extracted the active principle, purifying it, and modifying it to make it more active, longer lasting, less toxic, more controllable. Although many of these long-established drugs, like aspirin for instance, are now produced synthetically, digitalis is still made from foxgloves – but not now from the familiar purple variety.

This method of hunting for drugs has by no means been abandoned. In mid-1984 a team was reported to be trying to find the ingredient in green bananas that seems to have a powerful effect in preventing stomach ulcers. But during the 1960s and '70s a different approach has produced a number of new groups of drugs. One of them was a group called beta blockers.

Beta blockers

The first beta blocker was found as the result of a hunt for a drug to treat angina, the pain that gives warning of the possibility of a heart attack. The heart muscle, like any other muscle, needs a sufficient supply of oxygen to keep it operating, and the harder the heart is being asked to work, the more oxygen it needs. Normally the heart receives plenty of blood through the coronary arteries, but they can become furred up inside, and when that happens they can barely cope with the oxygen needs of the resting heart, let alone when the demand is increased by exercise or stress of some other kind.

At first people looking for effective drugs aimed, very reasonably, at finding a way of increasing the oxygen supply to the heart by dilating the coronary arteries – relaxing the walls of the vessels to allow more blood through. Drugs were found that did dilate the coronary vessels, but the trouble was that they dilated other vessels as well which meant that the demand for oxygen increased, so the heart was back in trouble again. However, there was another way of looking at the problem. The root of the difficulty was a lack of balance between supply and demand. If it was difficult to increase supply, how about reducing demand? Was that possible?

Since the body has its own system for increasing the heart's activity, and hence the oxygen demand, when it is being called to action, and decreasing it again when the heat is off, James Black, a pharmacologist working with the British chemicals firm I.C.I. at that time decided to have a look at that system and see whether it was possible to interrupt it.

Many of the body's control systems work through chemical messengers, which operate by fitting into matching molecules called receptors and switching them on, as a key might switch on a piece of electrical equipment. Two of these messenger chemicals, adrenalin and noradrenalin, were known to have some effect on the heart and blood vessels, and between them they could achieve a complicated change. They caused the heart to speed up and contract more powerfully; they caused some blood vessels to constrict, and others to expand, so that more blood would go to the muscles and less to such temporarily unimportant parts as the digestive system.

It was mainly the speeding up of the heart Black wanted to interrupt, and he would have to do this by making a dummy key that would fit and block the receptor and prevent the chemical messenger from getting in and activating it. At the time he began his work there was evidence that there were two different receptors involved, called alpha and beta. There were alpha and beta receptors on the blood vessels, but only beta on the heart, so it was a blocker for the beta receptors that was needed.

Black therefore knew precisely what he wanted his drug to do, and he could test it out in the laboratory on the type of tissue he wanted it to affect: heart muscle. In fact, he and his colleagues were just beginning to look at chemicals which they thought might be approximately the right shape when they had a stroke of luck. They read a paper from a group involved in entirely different work reporting on a substance that blocked their efforts to relax tissue similar to the walls of blood vessels. This was just a nuisance to the publishers of the paper, but not to Black. It was known that one chemical acting on the alpha and beta receptors had opposite effects on different tissues, stimulating the heart while relaxing the blood vessels. If this substance, too, affected tissues in opposite ways, then it should also block the body's own efforts to speed up the heart. It did. It was the first beta blocker.

It was the first of many, because beta blockers turned out to be useful in an extremely common disease.

Blood pressure
There is some disagreement about precisely what counts as 'high' blood pressure, and even more about the level that needs to be treated. There is not really a figure for normal blood pressure in the same way as the normal temperature is 37°C (98.4°F). A blood pressure of more than 145/90 (the two figures represent the pressure first as the surge from the heart's pumping motion is felt, and then as it drops back before the next beat) is regarded as too high, but it can be much lower than that and still be normal. High blood pressure, even when it does not cause any symptoms, is regarded as dangerous, because it makes people much more vulnerable to strokes, heart disease and kidney failure. It is for this reason that some doctors feel that high blood pressure should be treated even when it is causing no immediate trouble, and if it is treated then beta blockers are a likely choice of drug.

Since receptors, and the chemical messengers that activate them, are involved in a vast range of the body's control mechanisms, receptor theory is now one of the foundations of drug research. It has led to the discovery of many drugs — not only blockers, but others, like the synthetic hormones, for instance — that will mimic the body's own messenger and switch on the receptor.

Making the medicine go down
It is an amazing thought that the pill has only been with us since the end of the last century — not *the* Pill, but the pill, the small disc-shaped object made of compressed powder in which so many of our common medicines are packaged. Until then, medicine usually came in bottles, and you had no choice but to taste the stuff. It was well known that the nastier it tasted the better it was for you.

The pill is a most convenient way of carrying and taking drugs, but in practice it is less than ideal because it is not predictable just when and where it will dissolve and deliver its contents to be absorbed. This can be more of a problem than it sounds, because a drug that is designed to be released and absorbed in one part of the digestive system may not be absorbed at all if it is released in the wrong place. On one occasion a consignment of ampicillin, normally a very effective antibiotic drug, was exported to Africa. Nobody could understand why it seemed to be useless at dealing with the infection it was aimed at, but near miraculous as a cure for constipation. It turned out that there was nothing wrong with the drug in the capsules. The powder in which it was contained had been over-compressed, which made it less porous. The tablets did not dissolve high up in the intestinal tract where they were supposed to, and where the drug would be absorbed into the system. Instead they were arriving more or less intact in the large intestine, where they killed off all the friendly bacteria that we all have living in our large intestine, hence the diarrhoea. The effectiveness of a pill depends on more than the strength and purity of the drug it contains.

As drugs have become more sophisticated, so have the containers in which they are served up. The new types of packaging have two principal aims: to control the time when the drugs are released and to control the place where they are released. Often the aim is to make it happen over as long a period as possible. One problem about drugs is that once they have dissolved and the body can get to work on them they may be eliminated very quickly, so frequent doses have to be taken. The best solution to that would be if the drug, having been taken in one dose, is made available to the body a little at a time.

The right time
Many ways of doing this have been found. Sometimes it can be done on the molecule of the drug itself. In insulin, for instance, a slow-acting form can be produced by attaching the insulin molecule to other proteins. This makes it less soluble, and so delays its action. But often the slow release is built into the delivery system rather than the drug. There is the familiar 'cold cure' type of capsule which consists of an outer coat of gelatin with hundreds of tiny capsules inside which all dissolve at different rates. This releases the drug slowly, but the rate at which it works depends on the contents of the stomach. With powerful drugs like some of the anti-inflammatory pain killers, where an effective dose is uncomfortably close to a dangerous one, the precise timing is more important, so in 1983 a new capsule was introduced as a once-a-day container for a well-established drug, indomethacin.

The container was a larger than average pill, in which the drug was enclosed in a porous membrane so that as soon as it reached the liquid environment of the stomach it would dissolve. However, while the pores in the membrane were large enough to let the liquid in, they were too small to let the dissolved drug out, so the only way out for the drug was through one single hole, precision drilled with a laser, which was still tiny, but large enough to allow the drug to trickle through very slowly. It looked like the perfect solution, but unfortunately it did not behave as predicted. Precisely why the pill failed was not clear, but there were reports of perforated ulcers and headaches, and so it was withdrawn. It was thought that the cause of the trouble might be the pill sticking and releasing all its drugs in one spot, destroying the protective mucus in the stomach; or alternatively it was suggested the cause might be the salt with which the drug was solidified causing irritation. Whatever the cause, *this* drug in *this* pill was a bad partnership and the makers withdrew it from the market. The drug itself is still available, but once again it has to be taken four times a day, and the pill is likely to be launched again soon, but holding a different drug, possibly a beta blocker.

Sometimes a drug must last not just a day or two, but for much longer, and then the solution is different. Drugs can be trapped into oily liquids, gels, and solid lumps of material which can be either injected or implanted. These can be designed so that the drugs will diffuse out slowly and evenly over days, months, even years. These methods of delivering drugs may be useful for cancer drugs and contraceptives, and, in Third World countries particularly, for infectious diseases where it is important that treatment is continued for a long period.

A sticking plaster to treat heart disease sounds like a bad joke, but it is nothing of the kind. Although the skin is an excellent protective coat, it does allow some materials to pass across it. We can lose up to 2 litres – about 4 pt – a day through our sweat glands, and while the skin would certainly not allow in 2 litres of rain, it will allow some materials to pass inwards. One of the first occasions when this was seen to be happening was during the Second World War when munitions workers began to suffer from headaches, and it was discovered that they were absorbing chemicals from the explosives they were handling through their skins. In the same way, the chemicals contained in some drugs will diffuse through the skin. This might be an ideal way of taking them if the drug could be applied to this skin continuously and in a controlled way. Hence the sticking plaster. In place of the gauze pad that normally sits on the inside of a wound dressing, these sticking plasters have a layer of drug, sometimes contained in a gel or oily liquid, covered with a membrane. This membrane is necessary because skin is not reliable. The rate at which it can absorb chemicals can vary a great deal, whereas the membrane allows the drug to diffuse through at a precise rate. It is particularly ingenious because it is composed of two different types of polymer (long chain molecules) and by changing the proportions of the two types in the mix the membrane can be made more or less permeable. The first of these sticking plasters to be developed contained a heart drug, a more recent one holds a drug to combat seasickness.

The right place
There are times when the important consideration is not when a drug is absorbed but where. One way of directing drugs to a particular target is by attaching them to specific antibodies (see page 00), but other strategies rely on delivering the drugs in parcels of a particular size, and made of particular material.

The liposome is a packet composed of a sort of man-made copy of a cell membrane. When used as a drug container, it can either be a tiny envelope, or it can be multi-layered like an onion, with the drug interspersed in or between the layers, so that it will diffuse out slowly layer by layer. Because it is covered in a membrane similar to a cell's the liposome is not broken down quickly, as a simple chemical might be,

OPPOSITE A technician installs the equipment which carried out the first experiments in the purification of drugs in space during a 1984 space shuttle flight

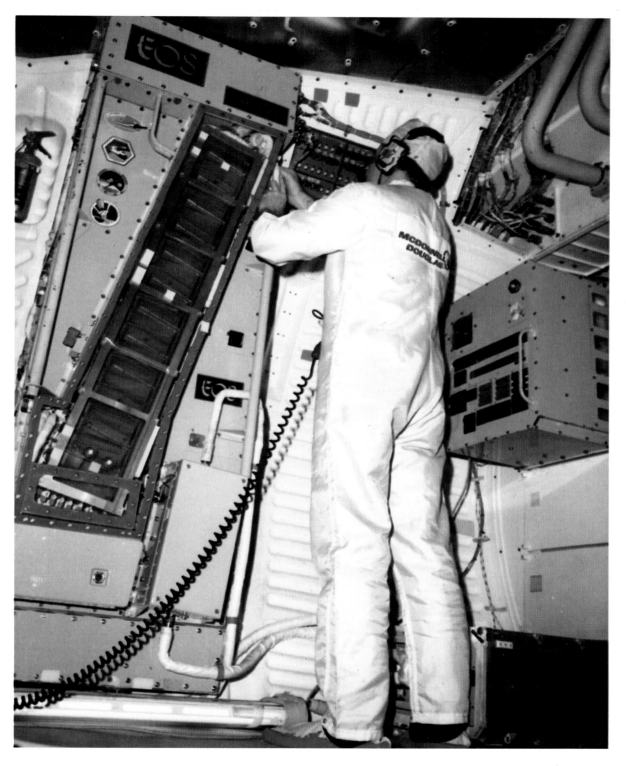

but travels round the body for some time. However, since the liposomes
lack the protein markers that might identify them to the body as 'self',
the macrophages, cells involved in the immune reaction, treat them as

foreign and swallow them, and in practice this results in most of the drug being released in the liver and spleen. One of the most successful uses of liposomes so far has been in the treatment of Leishmaniasis, a tropical infectious disease. The organisms that cause the disease congregate in the liver and spleen, and when the drug that kills these organisms is delivered wrapped in liposomes it is 200 times as effective as on its own.

A more recent development, which is still at the experimental stage, uses red cells instead of the artificial membrane. The cells are removed from the blood, emptied of their contents and filled with the appropriate drug. If group O blood is used, then the drug-filled cells can be injected into a member of any blood group without ill effects. This system has been shown to be effective in delivering steroid drugs to inflamed joints, and there are also plans to try the system with other medicines, including cancer drugs.

Both liposomes and red cells will travel round the body until they are taken up by macrophages. Attempts are also being made to find a way of creating a drug packet that can be absorbed by other types of cell, in the same way as they absorb nutrients. This work too is still experimental, but it seems that by attaching a drug to one end of a long chain molecule, and a protein that is absorbed by liver cells at the other end, it should be possible to create a drug that will be taken up by liver cells, perhaps to treat liver cancer.

Production
Until very recently the drug manufacturer had two broad options. Either he could extract his drug from a source in nature, or he could build it up from simple chemicals. Sometimes drugs that had originally been found in nature could be made synthetically, but the usual rule was that simple compounds were made synthetically, and complicated ones would come from plants. But some substances which are very useful in medicine cannot easily be made by either method. They are the enzymes and hormones which are too complicated to be built up from simple chemicals, but are very difficult to extract from the small quantities of human or animal cells available. In the production of these compounds advances in biotechnology promise to make an enormous difference.

Biotechnology
There is nothing new about biotechnology itself. Beer, wine and yoghurt are all products of biotechnology. What is new is the introduction into the field of the techniques of genetic engineering. The transformation took place when it was discovered it was possible to take a gene that carried the information necessary to make a chemical which is vital to man, to insert it in among the genetic material of a single-celled organism like a bacterium or yeast, and then to put it into a fermenting

tank in which it would multiply and produce a plentiful supply of the desirable chemical, which could be filtered off from the production line at intervals.

As a result of genetic engineering, human insulin made by bacteria is now an alternative to the usual supplies made from the pancreatic cells of cows or pigs. Interferon, too, is being produced this way, and a string of other human hormones, enzymes and other proteins.

Human production lines

Bacteria are used instead of human cells in this type of process because, unlike bacteria and yeasts, animal cells do not grow happily floating around in a broth; they prefer something solid to sit on. One exception to this is in the production of monoclonal antibodies (see page 00), but they involve the use of cancer cells, and one difference between normal and cancer cells is that the latter are less dependent on a fixed base. Recent work suggests that it may be possible to solve this difficulty by growing animal or human cells on tiny droplets of oil, or sponges or beads, suspended in a solution of nutrients, and this may extend the number of medically useful products that can be made by these living production lines.

Drugs from outer space

When the Apollo space missions returned to earth they brought moon rocks. Space shuttlers now are more likely to bring something that has a more immediately obvious use to man – drugs. It seems incredible, but there are drug companies who believe that some of their products can be made so much more efficiently away from the 'nuisance' of gravity that it will be worth their while in the future to buy facilities in space labs and on shuttles.

It is not really the manufacture of the drugs that is being tried in space, but their purification, by a method known as continuous flow electrophoresis. The purification is done inside a column where a buffer solution is flowing upwards (this is on earth, where there *is* an upwards) in a steady stream. At the bottom of the stream the mixture to be separated out into its component parts is injected. Each different type of molecule is likely to have a different charge, so when an electric current is applied across the stream the molecules will be deflected away from the centre to varying degrees. By the time the material reaches the top it will consist of a number of separate streams that can be taken off and used. On earth this method works very imperfectly, because gravity can distort the flow, and because of gravity convection currents can arise in the buffer solution, which upsets the result. The first tests of the process in space, with no gravity to confuse the issue, suggest that it may be possible to complete the process 700 times as quickly, and produce drugs that are 4 times as pure. If results like that are confirmed on a larger scale then it may even be worth risking space sickness for them.

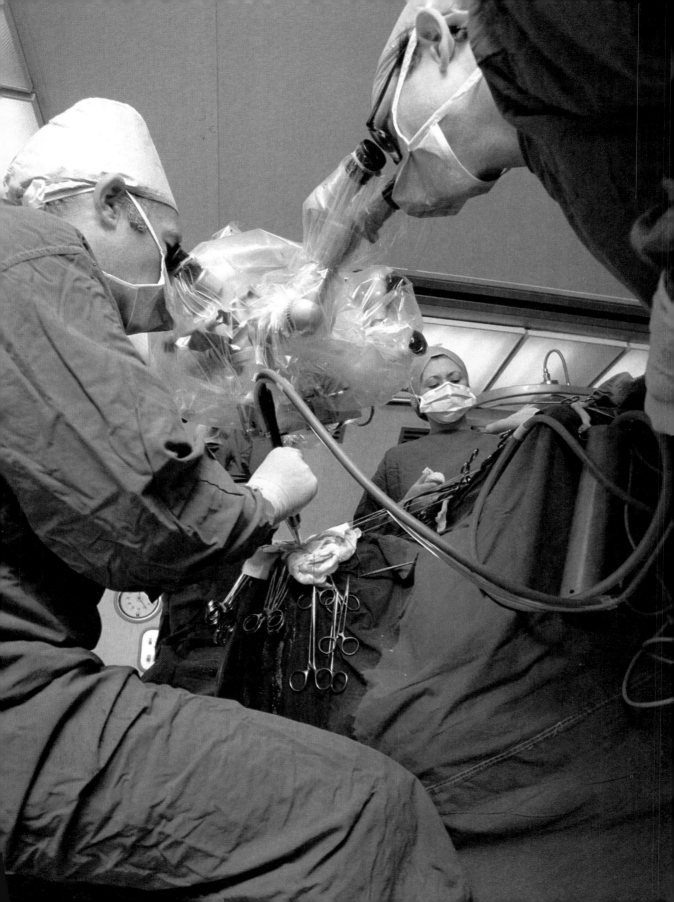

CHAPTER FIVE

Surgery

Scalpel and stitch as the beginning and end of surgery are still the rule rather than the exception – but only just. For many purposes the scalpel has given way to the laser, and occasionally the cryoprobe. And there are surgeons who would replace catgut with sticky tape, or even glue.

Lasers

There are half a dozen different types of laser in use in medicine, but only three are widespread. A laser (*Light Amplification by Stimulated Emission of Radiation*) produces an intense parallel beam of light energy of a particular wavelength or colour. The wavelength depends on the type of molecule that is being stimulated to emit the light. In medicine the three most common ones are carbon dioxide, argon and Neodymium yttrium-aluminium-garnet, understandably always known as either YAG or, to purists, Nd YAG.

Naturally enough the effect of a laser on tissue depends on how powerful it is. At the lowest energies it does no more than warm the target; as it gets stronger it shrinks and hardens tissue (rather like the effect of the heat of the grill on bacon); and at full power it chars or vaporizes. The beam of a laser can be focused very finely, to a spot of less than a thousandth of a millimetre, and when it is used at high power moving back and forth over a line it cuts as a scalpel, but even so there will be some lower-energy effect on the surrounding tissue. So where a laser is used to cut, the tissue immediately alongside will be shrunk and hardened (just like the bacon), and this has the highly desirable effect of contracting the cut ends of any tiny blood vessels, closing them off. Alternatively, if the target itself is a bleeding ulcer the laser may be used at lower power purely for this hardening and coagulating effect.

The light emitted from each of the lasers used in medicine is in a different part of the spectrum. The carbon dioxide's is in the middle of the infra-red portion, the argon in the visible blue-green, and the YAG in the near infra-red. The fact that the emission from each laser is at a specific wavelength is very important, because it means that each affects the tissue in a different way.

Carbon dioxide: CO_2 laser light is very effectively absorbed by water, and since tissue can consist of up to 90 per cent water, 98 per cent of the energy of a CO_2 beam is absorbed in the first hundredth of a millimetre of tissue. Surgical carbon dioxide lasers are quite powerful, typically between 30 and 100 watts. One of their drawbacks is that at the moment the light cannot be carried in an optical fibre, because its wavelength is absorbed by glass, quartz and other materials of which optical fibres can as yet be made.

Argon: Unlike the carbon dioxide laser, the argon laser travels straight through water. It is absorbed much more strongly by darker-coloured elements in the tissues, like the red cells of blood and the melanin that

Microsurgeons at work on the brain, using an ultrasound probe to liquefy and remove a tumour, see page 82 colours skin exposed to strong sunlight. Argon lasers are less powerful than carbon dioxide, up to about 15 watts, but they have the advantage that they can be carried on optical fibres.

Neodymium – YAG: This is not absorbed in water anything like as efficiently as the carbon dioxide laser, nor is it particularly well absorbed in darker pigments. It therefore tends to penetrate and heat tissue more deeply than the other two. Medical Nd YAG lasers are powerful, up to 100 watts, and they can be carried on optical fibres. Because the energy of the argon laser is absorbed particularly in pigmented tissue, that is the laser used in the most common and best established of all laser treatments.

Diabetic blindness

The commonest cause of blindness starting in the middle years in Britain is diabetes. One long-term result of diabetes is damage to tiny blood vessels all over the body. This complication can be particularly serious in the retina, the surface at the back of the eye which contains the rods and cones that convert the 'picture' entering the eye into signals, and in the nerves that convey those signals to the brain. The retina is criss-crossed with a network of minute blood vessels. When these are damaged by diabetes the whole retina is starved of blood. It reacts by producing a chemical that causes abnormal growth of blood vessels through the surface of the retina, which then becomes scarred and distorted and finally tears apart, resulting in total blindness. In the past there was very little that could be done to stop this happening, but with the advent of the laser, doctors feel it should be possible to prevent that final disaster befalling at least 85 per cent of those whose symptoms are noticed early.

The reason why the argon laser is able to help is that the top layer of the retina, which covers the rods and cones, is quite a dark colour; it is called the pigment layer. The beam of the argon laser shines through the lens of the eye on to any affected parts of the surface. The light is absorbed, converted to heat, and destroys this pigment layer. If this is done as soon as the first signs of damage to the eye can be seen then there is no production of the chemical that causes the abnormal growth. Since light at this wavelength is also absorbed by the blood cells, the laser can equally well be used to treat any abnormal blood vessels that are already developing. The burning away of the surface does do some damage to the eyesight – particularly colour vision – but in the vast majority of people it is able to stop the progress towards total blindness.

This is obviously a task that could never be performed with a knife, however skilfully handled. In eye surgery the laser is also used – this time the more powerful YAG – to substitute for the knife, to cut out the lens in cataract, and to improve drainage to release the pressure of glaucoma.

Skin blemishes

'Be tattooed in haste and repent at leisure' could be an even more appropriate warning than the original proverb. A tattoo is more permanent than many a modern marriage. The old girl friend's name tattooed over the heart can be a considerable embarrassment when one or both have decided they are not after all the perfect couple. Or it may simply be that the tattoo owner's aesthetic sense changes. The ink of the tattoo is firmly embedded under the outer layer of the skin, the epidermis, in the top of the inner layer, the dermis, and it is not easily removed. Another skin blemish, this time occurring naturally, is the port wine stain. This is caused by a network of tiny transparent blood vessels immediately below the outer layer of the skin, and it is particularly distressing because it very frequently appears on the face. As its name implies, it can be very darkly coloured, almost purple, and very difficult to hide.

Because they can do so much damage to the self-image of the victim, all kinds of attempts have been made to find a treatment. Abrasion of the skin, ultraviolet radiation, surgery, skin grafting, even tattooing with a paler colour, all have been tried - and mostly abandoned; so until the laser, cosmetics were the only aid.

The argon laser looked like the perfect answer to both the port wine stain and the unwanted tattoo. The light should pass through the outer, colourless layer of the skin and be absorbed in the coloured ink of the tattoo or the red blood causing the port wine stain. The heat would either coagulate the blood vessels, or in the case of the tattoo break up the ink particles so that they were small enough to be cleared away by macrophages, the army of large cells which travel around the body swallowing and removing any debris.

In practice it does not work quite as ideally as that. The effect on the blood vessels and ink particles is much as expected, but there is quite severe burning of the skin. However, the skin regrows, usually without serious scarring, and despite slight disappointment this is regarded by some people as the best solution to the problem.

A kinder cut

The cervical smear campaign is the only widespread screening programme for the detection of early cancer. Samples of cells are scraped off the cervix, the neck of the womb, for examination to see whether there is any sign of the type of change in the cells that is regarded as a warning that cancer is likely to develop. When such cells are found then immediate treatment is needed, and the laser has many advantages over the knife. Using an operating microscope to distinguish between affected and healthy cells, a laser beam can be easily directed on to the surface of the cervix. It is easier than gaining access with a knife, and there are no instruments in the way to obstruct the view of the target. If the pre-cancer cells are not all accessible directly, then the beam can be

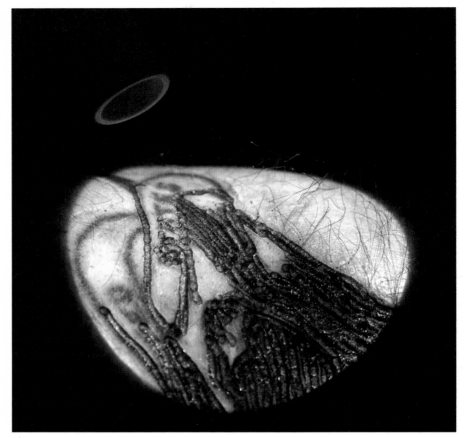

LEFT Unwanted tattoos can sometimes be removed by laser beams

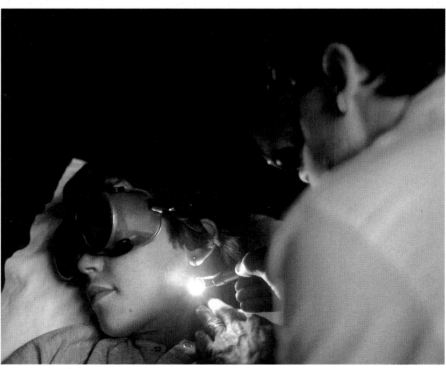

LEFT An argon laser at work removing a portwine stain

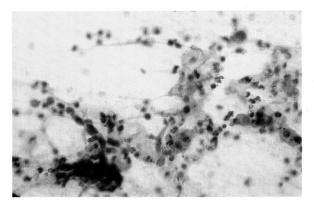 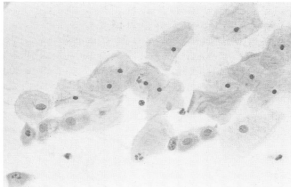

Two results of tests for cervical cancer. The first is of healthy cells, the other slide has cells which show signs of cancer

reflected at an angle through a mirror. The carbon dioxide laser is used, scanning across the affected area, vaporizing the tissue layer by layer until all the affected cells have been removed, together with any extra material that may be doubtful. If there is a need to provide a sample of tissue for laboratory examination, then the beam can be used as a knife, sealing any blood vessels it meets as it cuts, although if they are particularly large ones it may be necessary to defocus the laser and coagulate a larger volume of tissue to slow down the bleeding.

Lasers have only been in use in medicine for about ten years, and already they are employed to treat hundreds of different problems, although there is still an enormous amount to be found out. Not all tissues behave in the same way when bombarded with laser beams, and it is not always easy to predict how a new laser procedure will work. Sometimes the results will be disappointing. It was thought at one time that laser treatment of some small but very malignant cancers might be possible. But it turned out that although the laser destroyed the tumour it did this so energetically that there was a danger of spreading the malignant cells to start new secondary tumours. Now a different idea is gaining ground of how lasers might attack cancer. This could use much less powerful laser light, but the cancer cells would be treated first.

Photosensitization

The idea of photosensitization is to use chemicals to make cancer cells more sensitive to light. It is a possibility that was suggested more than ten years ago. Since then it has been lurking in the background and is only now beginning to be studied seriously.

The chemical that is most often used for the purpose is a dye called haematoporphyrin derivative, always known as HPD; haematoporphyrin is the substance that makes the blood red. When the man-made HPD is injected into the bloodstream it is first of all taken up by all cells, normal or cancerous. Then over the following two or three days the dye disappears completely from normal tissue, but stays fixed in cancer cells.

When light – and in practice it would be laser light – is shone on the dye inside the cell, then the energy is absorbed and the dye becomes excited. Precisely what happens next is not completely certain, but it seems that the dye breaks up any neighbouring oxygen molecules which form part of the cell membrane. Singlet oxygen, as these broken oxygen molecules are called, is highly dangerous to cells. It tears open the outer membrane, and the contents are destroyed.

One particularly useful fact about HPD is that when the dye has been absorbed in cells you can see it; it fluoresces a bright red colour when lit with blue light. So it is possible to check before bombarding the cells with the more powerful laser light that the dye has disappeared from all the normal cells in the vicinity.

Cryosurgery
You can cut tissue, you can burn it, you can also freeze it, and for some purposes freezing appears to be better than anything else.

The idea of cryosurgery is to destroy abnormal or diseased tissue by freezing it until it dies. If the unwanted tissue is a simple little skin blemish like a wart, then sufficient cold can be produced either by touching it with a piece of solid CO_2 (the dry ice that keeps the ice cream frozen) or by dabbing with a cotton wool swab dipped in liquid nitrogen.

Over the last 20 years, however, cryosurgeons have been provided with a variety of sprays and probes which have meant that much more adventurous procedures can be tried. A spray of liquid nitrogen is useful if there is a large area to be frozen, but most cryosurgery is done with a cryoprobe. This is an insulated metal rod. Inside its tip, which of course is not insulated, liquid nitrogen is allowed to expand. This absorbs so much heat from the probe tip that the metal cools to a temperature as low as $-180°C$. In an alternative type of probe it is the expansion of pressurised nitrous oxide gas into a lower pressure chamber at the tip that freezes the probe. But this type will only reach $-70°C$.

All these instruments are much cheaper than lasers, but cost is by no means their only virtue. Destruction by freezing causes less scarring than destruction by laser, or for that matter by cutting with a knife. Removal of a wart or ulcer by freezing can leave virtually no scar at all. Nobody is quite sure why this is, but it probably happens because of the way freezing destroys the tissue. The damage is not done by sharp ice crystals piercing the cells and breaking up the tissue. It appears that as the tissue freezes ice crystals begin to form in the watery solution between the cells. The ice crystals take pure water out of the solution, which gets saltier and removes water by osmotic pressure from the cells themselves. This upsets the balance inside the cells and they are killed. Although this process destroys the cells it leaves a scaffolding of collagen, a fibrous molecule which is an important constituent of the structure of muscle, skin etc. This surviving framework of collagen means that instead of regrowing in a muddle - which is in effect what a scar is — the cells re-form in the correct orderly fashion.

Another virtue of freezing is that it really is painless, apart from slight discomfort as the tissue thaws. The first thing the cold does is to paralyse the nerves, although it does not destroy them completely so they do regrow. (The central nerves, in the spinal column and brain, do not regrow in the same way, which is why cryosurgery can be used to treat chronic pain.)

The most frequent use of the cryoprobe at the moment is to treat skin blemishes, both benign blemishes like warts and skin cancers, and in this type of work the lack of scarring is a real bonus. Among the skin blemishes that are candidates for cryosurgery are the port wine stains which are often treated by laser. It seems that freezing small blood vessels, such as those that produce these stains, causes them to clot, and they do not reopen when thawed unless the probe has been jerked while the tissue was frozen and brittle. Haemorrhoids, known to the millions who suffer from them as piles, are also caused by damaged blood vessels, and cryosurgery has been tried as a treatment for them. There are enthusiasts, and non-enthusiasts, and whether it will ever be more than an experiment is still uncertain.

In one unusual application the cryoprobe takes the place of forceps rather than knife. The standard treatment for cataract is to remove the lens of the eye, which has become opaque, and replace it with an implant or a contact lens. As anyone who has ever tried to let go of a

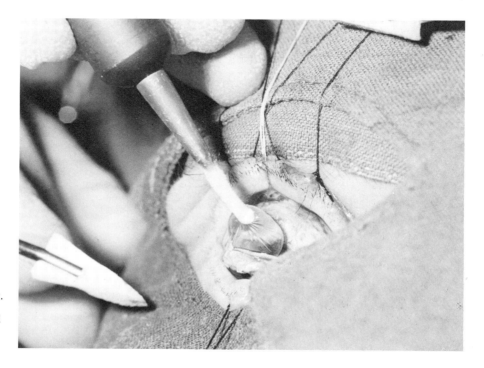

One way of treating cataract. The cloudy lens is removed from the eye, firmly gripped by the cold tip of the cryoprobe

really cold tray of ice cubes will know, a piece of frozen metal sticks very firmly to any wet, or even damp object. The same happens when the tip of a cryoprobe is applied to the lens of the eye. The probe holds the lens firmly, while it is loosened and removed. The grip between a cryoprobe and a wet surface like the lens of the eye has been tested, and it will lift a weight of at least 1 kg (2.2 lb).

Freezing will stop the passage of nerve signals long before the nerve is permanently damaged. This means that it is possible to try out the effect before any irreversible action. This was first exploited in brain surgery, but it can also be used in the heart.

Normally the electrical signals that control the heart are neatly arranged to pass from one half to the other in such a way that the filling and emptying is correctly synchronized. Sometimes that arrangement is upset, either by spare signals arising in the wrong place at the wrong time, or by something not unlike a short circuit. By freezing the tissue it is possible to destroy the abnormal connection; the only trouble is that it is not visible. But by chilling the likely spot first the surgeon can check that the unwanted signal has been stopped, and the heart is behaving properly, and only then freeze it thoroughly to destroy it completely.

There is one possibility about the effects of freezing tissue that could, if it is proved, increase the value of cryosurgery enormously. It is thought that after frozen tissue is thawed some components of the destroyed cells may be released into the bloodstream through vessels alongside the freeze. If the tissue being destroyed is a cancer, then these components might be characteristic of the cancer cells, and in the bloodstream they might act as a sort of vaccine, and stimulate an immune reaction, fighting not only any remaining cells close to the freeze, but also any cells from the tumour that have spread to other parts of the body. It is an exciting prospect, but so far there is only a very little rather inconclusive evidence that this effect exists. It may be that freezing in a slightly different way could help it along, but at the moment it has to be regarded as unproven.

Both lasers and cryoprobes are comparative newcomers to surgery, and it will take time to discover which is really the better tool for which task. There have been few, if any, large trials of one against the other. Removal of tumours is one thing for which both are being tried out, but for some neurosurgeons dealing with a particular type of tumour of the brain and spinal cord neither is the answer.

In 1983 the newspapers were full of stories of a little boy who had gone to New York to have a tumour removed from his spine with a wonderful new instrument. The instrument in question was in fact already in use in Britain in a number of NHS hospitals at the time. It is a probe which consists of a hollow titanium tube, with a tip that can be vibrated at ultrasonic frequency. When it is applied to the tumour the vibration emulsifies it, and it is sucked away. The virtue of this is that it removes the tissue gradually from the middle of the tumour, so that it collapses in on itself, and then it is possible to make room to pull the remainder away from the delicate structures surrounding it with much less risk of damaging them.

Whether some or all of these instruments will become a regular part of the equipment of every surgeon, or in the case of the cryoprobe perhaps also of every GP, only time and trial will tell. There seems to be very little doubt that both lasers and cryoprobes have a part to play in eye surgery. For the rest, if it is to be universally available, the laser will need to be a great deal cheaper and easier to maintain, and the relative merits of the different probes are still to be decided. Meanwhile, an individual surgeon's enthusiasm for a particular treatment will quite often depend principally on whether or not he has the necessary instrument at his disposal.

Surgery without scars

Any illness that can be successfully treated by surgery is, almost by definition, one where the basic fault is confined to one organ, or a small area of the body, even though its effects may be widespread. Yet although the surgeon's target may be very small, he often has to cause a lot of damage on his way to the faulty component. Lung surgery, for instance, has extremely painful after-effects not because the lungs are particularly sensitive, but because to get to the lung the surgeon has to cut his way through two layers of muscles and open the ribcage. Running inside the ribs are rows of tiny nerves, which can be pinched as the damaged muscles are brought back into play. Then the poor patient may

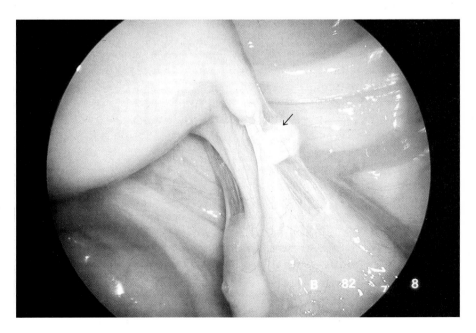

A ring obstructing the fallopian tube, one of a number of methods of sterilization which can be performed through a laparoscope

well begin to regard the physiotherapist (whose job it is to encourage surgical patients to rehabilitate themselves, and especially to exercise their chest and lungs) as a true descendant of the medieval torturers.

Because of these unpleasant after-effects for the patients, many doctors are making determined advances towards what might be described as minimal damage surgery. The aim is to find the way to the faulty component, and to correct it, with the least possible damage to the basic structure. Operations that once meant wounds almost as large as that for lung surgery are now being done through an endoscope, which may have been developed as a diagnostic aid but now has a complete tool kit for a more active role.

Gynaecologists and urologists probably make more active use of endoscopes than anyone else. Very few women would choose to have a sterilization if it meant they had to be cut widely open, but through a laparoscope a tiny incision allows the gynaecologist to cut and tie, seal or clip the fallopian tubes. (To open them up again takes a full-scale operation which is not always a success.)

Enlarged prostate is one of the most common disorders in older men; in fact nearly all men develop it to some degree, but it only becomes a real problem for about one in ten. The prostate is a gland, about the size of a walnut, where part of the seminal fluid is made. The gland sits immediately below the bladder, and as the enlargement grows it constricts the urethra making it difficult to pass water. Sufferers notoriously delay going to consult their doctor until it is causing at best inconvenience, at worst serious pain, often because they know a man who knew a man who died of the operation for enlarged prostate. So the operation gets a worse reputation because it is often left so late that it is almost an emergency; also the patients are often fairly elderly, making a general anaesthetic less desirable.

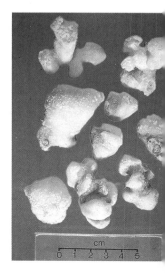

A choice selection of kidney stones of the staghorn type

Although the full operation is still quite common, most specialist urologists now remove enlarged prostates through a cystoscope passed through the urethra. The complete operation is done with a small wire loop on the end of a probe. A current is passed through the loop from a diathermy machine, which means that it not only cuts away the unwanted tissue, it also coagulates any tiny blood vessels which are damaged in the process. On the rare occasions when the trouble is caused by a cancer some kind of extra treatment is given and one course being tried out at the moment uses the endoscope to implant radioactive seeds in the remaining tissue to kill off any cancer cells.

The same endoscope that helps remove enlarged prostate has been used for years to remove bladder stones, but stones in the kidney present more of a problem.

Kidney stones

Kidney stones can form in different ways. Either they are due to an error of metabolism, usually the inability to handle calcium properly, in

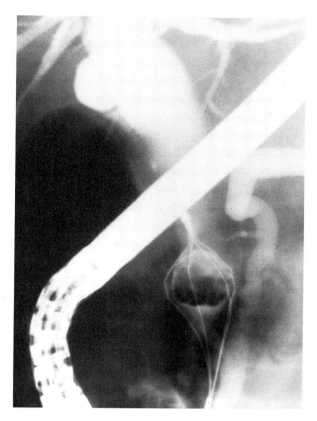

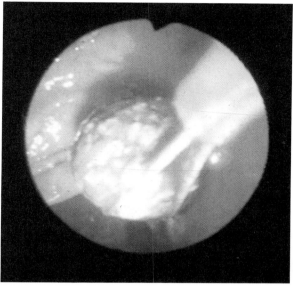

ABOVE LEFT X-ray view through the abdomen showing a gallstone gripped in a wire basket. The basket was pushed into the bile duct (from the tip of the endoscope just below the picture) folded inside a fine tube, and then opened up to grip the stone.

ABOVE RIGHT Endoscopic view. The stone still gripped in the basket has been pulled out of the bile duct and is now held in the duodenum

which case the stone grows from a tiny seed, rather like a pearl in an oyster. Alternatively they may be due to infection, in which case a sort of thick gel forms inside the kidney, making a mould of its interior. Later it solidifies into what is known as a staghorn calculus. A small stone may cause very little trouble for some of the time, but as it rolls about it can become wedged in one branch of the collecting system, the network of tubes inside the kidney. If the entry to that particular branch is blocked then urine can build up behind it and it becomes distended. Or worse, a stone can become wedged in the ureter, damming up the whole system. The one thing that makes the sensory nerves in the walls of vessels like these react violently is being stretched, so this sort of blockage is excruciatingly painful.

There are two possible ways to reach a kidney stone through an endoscope. The first is by using the body's normal passageways, through the urethra, bladder and ureter. The problem of that approach is that it is only possible to see into the top of the kidney, and the inner cavity of the kidney has many branches in which a stone can hide. The only way to gain access to the majority of these cavities, known as calices, is by making a forced entry through a hole in the side of the lower back. With the help of X-ray pictures the way to the kidney is found with a needle, and then the hole is gradually stretched until it is wide enough for the nephroscope (kidney endoscope).

When the stone is found – and even when it has been seen on the X-ray that can be quite difficult – the next stage depends on its size. If it is small enough it may be grabbed with a pair of jaws: a sort of remote-controlled crocodile clip. Or it may be gathered into a rather ingenious basket. But very frequently the stone is too big to remove in one piece and it needs to be broken up with ultrasound, shock waves, or even with a laser.

It is only about three years since this technique of treating kidney stones through endoscopes was developed. Yet already it may be becoming obsolete because of a new development which has recently come from Germany, affectionately known as the big banger, or extra-corporeal shock-wave lithotriptor. This breaks up stones with a shock wave, but does it remotely through the body tissue without making contact with the stone.

The owner of the offending kidney stone(s) is immersed up to the neck in a bath of water. One person in four has a general anaesthetic, but most people find that they can face it with only the epidural type of local pain block. The 'gun' that fires the shock waves at the stone is fixed in the bottom of the bath. It consists of a pair of electrodes mounted in an ellipse-shaped cup. The electrodes are positioned at one focus of the

BELOW The 'big banger' or extracorporeal shock wave lithotripter in use
INSET All reflected shock waves are focussed on the kidney stone when it is correctly positioned

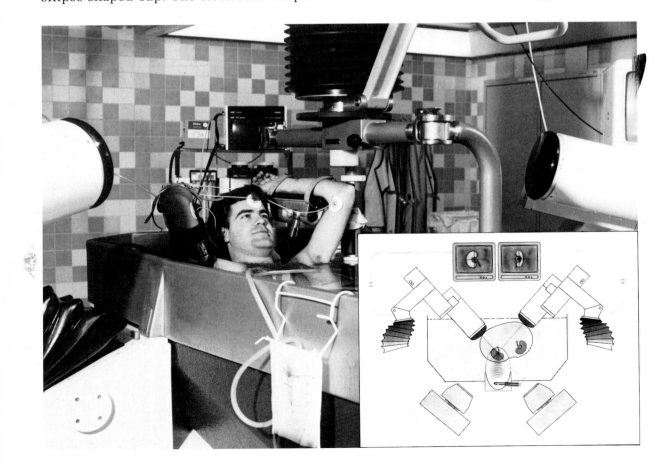

ellipse, and the effect of this particular shape is that both the original wave and the reflections from the sides of the cup are all directed on to the second focus of the ellipse; so that is where the stone has to be positioned. The patient is sitting in a hydraulically operated support so this is manoeuvred into more or less the right place, and then two X-ray cameras set at right angles to one another are used to make sure the stone is at precisely the right point. Then they are ready for firing.

When the electrode is fired, the shock waves pass through the water and the watery tissue quite harmlessly. It is only when they come up against an abrupt change of density, like the change from tissue to stone, that they have their shattering effect. It takes more than one shock to disintegrate a stone, hundreds in fact. In Germany, where the technique was developed, they give them in batches of 100. If the stone has not been demolished by the time they have given 1500 then they stop for the time being and give a second, or even a third treatment.

When the developers first began this type of treatment in 1980 they ran into an awkward problem. The shocks were interfering with the heart's electrical system causing quite severe disturbances in the patient's heartbeat. They found they could solve this by making sure that the shock was always given at a particular point in the heart's cycle. The simple way of making sure of that was to link up the patient's ECG (the electrical pattern of the heart) to the machine, and get the heartbeat to trigger the spark, and that is how it is done now.

Not all kidney stones are accessible to the big banger. Because the shock waves will have their effect whenever they meet a change of density in the substance they are passing through, it is very important not to hit the lungs, which will be full of air. So the waves must be aimed at the kidney between the bottom of the lungs and the top of the hip bone, and if the kidney is very high up it may be difficult to avoid the lungs. A few other stones are so tough that they will not break, even with thousands of shock waves, and others are so large that the resulting fragments would pack the kidney too tightly to wash away. But apart from these specially awkward ones, many experts think that in the not too distant future all kidney stones should be treatable this way, and that open surgery will be necessary in no more than a handful of cases.

The makers of the big banger are now looking at the possibility of dealing in the same way with the other common type of stone, the gallstone. That would be particularly valuable because gallstones are not always accessible by endoscope.

New tools, new prospects
The possibilities of endoscopic surgery depend very much on the type of tools that have been developed. There were difficulties in creating a suitable cryoprobe (the tip tended to take too long to freeze and thaw, and cold damaged the endoscope), but these have now been overcome; and lasers can be used with both flexible and rigid 'scopes. The lasers

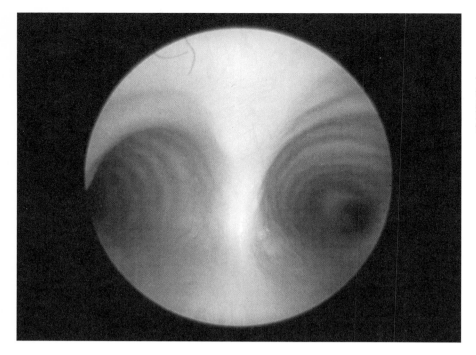

The carina, the point where the two lungs are joined. Laser surgery may be the best way of treating a tumour in this area

have not been available long enough for the best routines to be worked out, and until they are nobody will know when they are useful and when they are not. But one potential use is in treating bleeding from the digestive tract. Nearly 30,000 people a year are admitted to hospital as emergencies because of this type of bleeding, which is often due to an ulcer in the stomach, and trials are being conducted to see whether lasers can help, using the 'frying bacon' effect.

Another hopeful area is in the treatment of tumours in the oesophagus or lung. These are particularly horrible because the sufferer can starve to death or suffocate, and the laser is being used to cut away part of the tumour and open up a passage. One common position for a lung tumour is the place where the airways to the two lungs divide, called the carina because it looks like the prow of a boat. This is exceptionally difficult to deal with since lung surgery normally means removal of the affected part of the lung, and this part obviously cannot be removed. However, a laser used through a bronchoscope may be able to cut away the most obstructive part of the tumour, which would not be a cure, but would allow the patient to breathe. This treatment is difficult at the moment because the best 'knife' laser, the carbon dioxide type, cannot be used through a flexible endoscope, so it may have to wait until a fibre is developed that can carry the CO_2 laser beam.

Long-range surgery
Doctors using endoscopes usually aim at finding the shortest practicable route from the fresh air to their site of operations, but there is another range of procedures which uses the body's own underground system, the blood vessels, to travel from one part to another. Medical or surgical treatments of many kinds can be carried out through an inci-

sion 5 mm (0.2 in) long, often made at the opposite end of the body from the target.

In this sort of procedure a long thin tube known as a catheter is inserted into a blood vessel at a convenient point. The most common entry point on the red, arterial line (see illustration page 00) is in the groin, where the femoral artery is just below the surface. The femoral artery is a large artery which supplies the leg with blood: you can feel your own pulsing if you press at the point marked on the 'map'. There is a similar access to the blue, venous line, in the groin, since the femoral vein is large and leads straight into the vena cava, the body's most important vein. The carotid artery and jugular vein in the neck are other popular access points.

The doctors providing this form of treatment are usually radiologists rather than surgeons, because the route of the catheter through the blood vessels is found with the help of X-rays.

Since the blood vessels go everywhere, one obvious use for this technique is to deliver a dose of drugs to precisely the right part of the body, but there are other much less obvious ways that a cleverly steered catheter can be used to perform 'surgery'.

Heart disease is second only to cancer as a cause of death in Britain and many other industrialized nations. Some of the reasons for the large numbers who succumb to heart disease are now becoming clear, but until we can be persuaded to change some aspects of our life style the medical profession is going to have to pick up the pieces, and this long-range 'surgery' via X-ray-guided catheters can help.

The heart is a lump of highly active muscle, which needs a good supply of oxygen to keep going. It gets this through an array of small arteries which run down on the outside of the heart, being fed directly from the aorta, the main artery. In coronary heart disease these small arteries gradually become blocked with a fatty deposit called atheroma, and the heart finds itself inadequately supplied with blood. This causes pain, known as angina, and if the artery becomes severely narrowed, or even totally blocked by a small clot getting wedged in a narrowed section, then a heart attack is the catastrophic result.

Angina can often be treated with drugs, but if the arteries are very badly furred, and particularly if the blockage is in one of the two principal coronary arteries, then surgery is usually recommended. This is the well-known coronary bypass operation, undergone by a procession of the famous, in which small sections of vein are grafted on to carry blood past the blockages in the coronary arteries. The operation involves opening up not only the chest but also the leg, because that is where the sections of vein come from.

In the long-range alternative a catheter, which has a wire inside to steer it, is fed from the femoral artery up the aorta and into the coronary artery at the top. The catheter is pushed through past the narrowed part, and then the wire is withdrawn, leaving the tube in position. Through

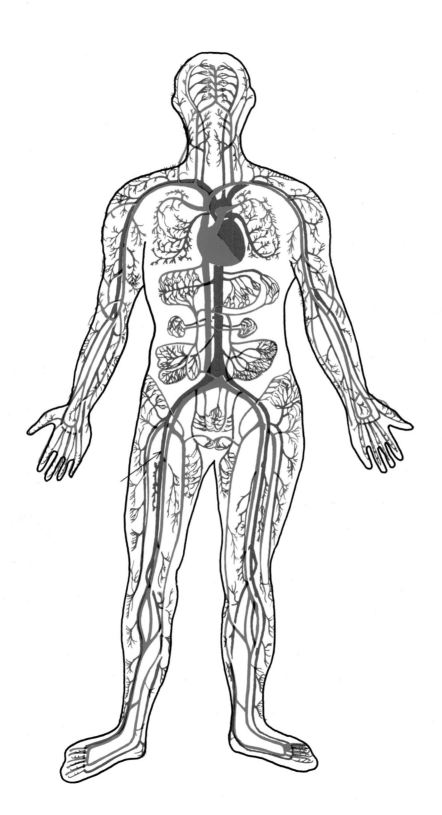

LEFT The map of the major blood vessels. Almost every vessel shown here can be reached by feeding a tube into the femoral artery or vein

BELOW A surgical procedure in progress with the help of pictures from a DVI x-ray machine

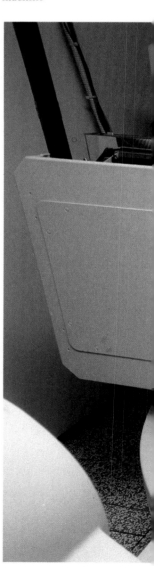

the catheter is fed a smaller tube which has an uninflated sausage-shaped balloon at its tip, and when that is in position the outer catheter is withdrawn, and the balloon is gently blown up with a syringeful of a solution that will show up on an X-ray. The length of time it can be held inflated varies from heart to heart, since the balloon itself will temporarily block the artery. It may be 15 seconds; it may be 3 minutes before the heart protests and blood must be allowed through. If it is only 15 seconds then it will be necessary to repeat the procedure.

There are different views about why the artery stays stretched when the balloon is withdrawn, but it seems likely that more than one change in the vessel is made by the balloon. First the deposit inside the vessel is

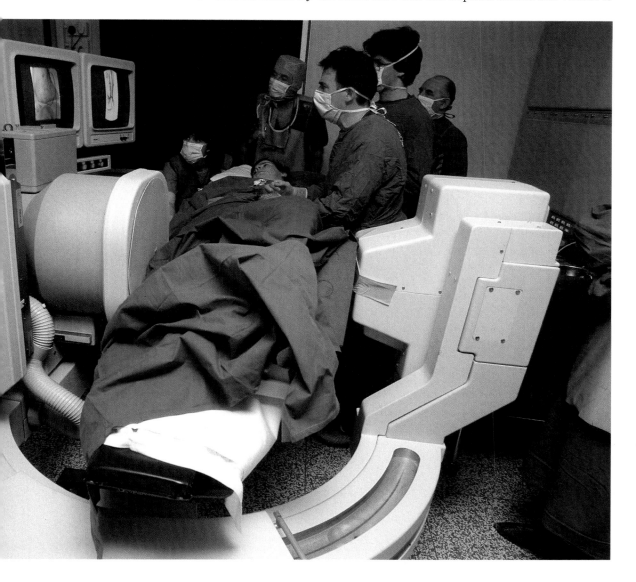

squashed flat. It is even suggested that this flattening breaks it down in some way so that the blood is able to wash some of the components away. But probably much more important is the fact that the balloon breaks down the elastic structure of the vessel wall, making it 'baggy'.

If a balloon can be fed through a catheter in this way, then so can an optical fibre, carrying a laser beam. If the beam is directed at the fatty deposits then it should be able to vaporize them so that the remains can be washed away in the bloodstream. The chief danger in this idea is that in the process tiny fragments of the deposit could be dislodged and pass on to block smaller vessels completely, and nobody knows yet whether or not this will happen. Yet another alternative is to use the catheter to inject a chemical called streptokinase, which is a natural substance used to break down fibrin, one of the constituents of blood clots.

The coronary arteries, too, may have their equivalent of the kidney stone 'big banger'. It is a treatment designed to work by remote control, although this one does involve an injection. The idea is to melt the fatty deposit. First a solution of tiny magnetic particles is injected into the bloodstream. The atheroma is much more permeable than normal arterial walls, so the particles should collect there more than anywhere else. Then the patient is put inside a large induction coil and subjected to a high-frequency electromagnetic field. This should react with the particles, producing heat to melt the fat. Unlike the kidney stone banger, this treatment is still very much at the experimental stage.

It will probably be some years before all these methods have been tested well enough for anyone to tell whether they should take over from current treatments. The coronary bypass operation has a good safety record and these newer techniques have yet to prove themselves in any but a few highly skilled hands.

Embolization

There are a few people who do not have the choice between these new techniques and the established ones. For them there is no established treatment, and it is the possibility of helping them that the radiologists find most exciting about these developments.

In 1982 a girl called Avril appeared in the BBC *Tomorrow's World* programme (the two X-rays on page 000 are hers). At the time when the first was taken she described herself as 'looking like an American footballer – all padded up'. Avril had a large tumour growing at the top of her arm. Even though it was not a cancer, and therefore would not spread to another part of her body, the doctors still told her that the only solution was to have the arm amputated. Avril refused point-blank, and as a last resort she came to see one of the pioneers of interventional radiology, as these treatments are called. He decided that there was a good chance of helping to save Avril's arm by starving the invader. As a tumour grows it sets up its own network of blood vessels, diverting the blood supply away from the surrounding tissues in the process. In

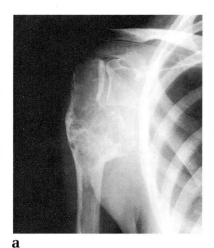
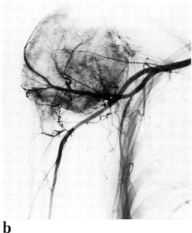
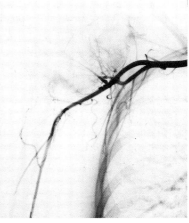

a   b   c

(a) X-ray of a shoulder of a girl with a tumour
(b) Similar view, but with bones subtracted and blood vessels only visible, showing the tumour with its blood supply.
(c) After vessels feeding the tumour are blocked it is starved of blood and disappears

A coil used for blocking arteries. While it is manoeuvred into position it is stretched out straight in the tube on the right. As it is pushed out of the tube it springs automatically into this shape.

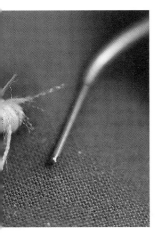

Avril's case that meant that the bone at the top of her arm was receiving very little blood and was wasting away. A surgeon might well be able to cut the main vessel feeding the tumour, but when that is done the blood nearly always manages to find its way into the tumour's branching vessels by another route. Smaller vessels merely increase their flow to compensate. An alternative is to make a much more substantial block, not only of the main vessel but of many of the smaller branches as well, and that needs to be done from inside the vessels. In Avril's case the blocking was done by threading a catheter through her arteries to the point where the vessels branched to feed the tumour, and then injecting a mixture of a type of foam sponge, stiffened with fragments of a substance called dura mater, the tough membrane that covers the brain and spinal cord. Since the early 1980s a range of materials has been tried out as blocks for blood vessels, and as a last resort even a plug of superglue can be used. A favourite now, however, is a small stainless-steel coil, coated in a sort of cotton material which induces the blood itself to form a clot and block the vessel in a more natural way. Blocking of blood vessels in this way is not only done to starve tumours; it can also be very useful in stopping bleeding – as from a deep stab wound.

The range of applications for this minimally invasive surgery is expanding all the time, and it is not easy to predict its limitations. One user of the techniques, challenged that it would never be possible to remove an appendix this way, was not defeated. 'Well,' he said, 'possibly you could use a flexible endoscope. You could go up inside the gut, turn the appendix inside out into the caecum [the point where the small intestine joins the large], then you could tie or staple it, and cut it off and remove it.' That particular approach may or may not be possible, but one surgeon has already developed a method of removing the appendix through three tiny incisions one for viewing and two for tubes through which scissors, forceps and needles can be manipulated.

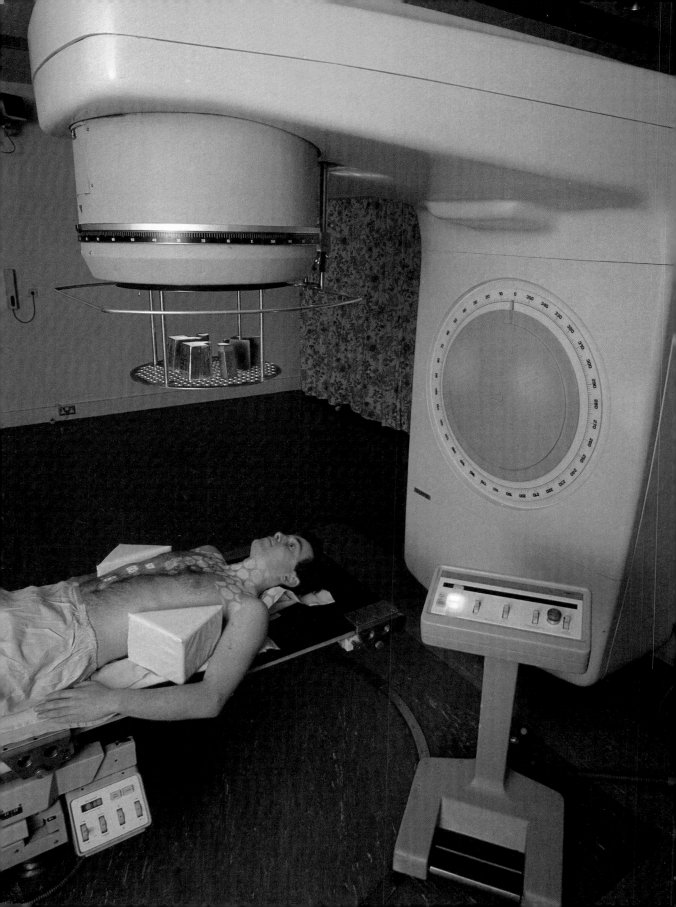

Radiation

At the same time as X-rays were demonstrating their usefulness in diagnosis by helping in the location of bullets and lumps of shrapnel buried in the flesh of soldiers wounded in the First World War, early trials were beginning on another use of radiation. Scientists who had put their hands too often in the path of the rays had noticed that they had an effect on the skin, and this had sparked the idea that they might be useful in treatment.

At first the exciting rays were used to treat a large variety of different complaints, arthritis and neuritis, eczema, ringworm and other skin troubles, as well as cancer. The treatment was very effective, both in relieving pain and in banishing the skin damage, although there were worrying signs that while the radiation could cure cancer it also seemed to be able to cause it. At first these cancers caused by radiation only appeared in people who were working continuously with the rays, or with radioactive materials. Then in Israel a group of immigrants who had been treated for ringworm, a legacy from their time in Nazi concentration camps, began to develop skin cancers. A few cases of leukaemia also appeared in people treated with radiation for a crippling bone disease called ankylosing spondylitis. Since the link was established between these cancers and the radiation therapy it has been reserved for use almost exclusively in the treatment of malignant disease – cancer.

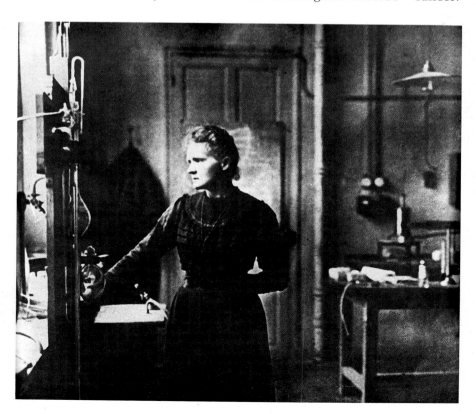

RIGHT Marie Curie, discoverer of radioactive elements including radium

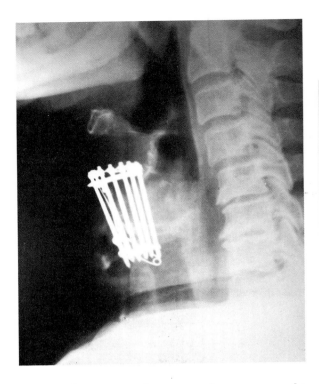

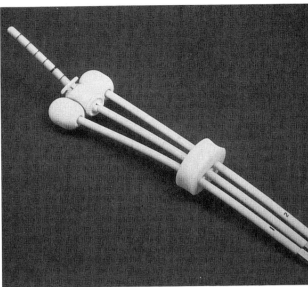

At the beginning the same tubes were used to produce X-rays both for diagnosis and for treatment. This proved unsatisfactory; the rays were of low power, and at treatment levels they caused too much skin damage. By the early 1920s other sources of the ionizing radiation were being introduced. Radium, or sometimes radon, the gas given off by radium, was enclosed in tiny platinum needles, which were implanted into the tumour and surrounding tissue. Early reports of the result were very enthusiastic, and Marie Curie, the discoverer of radium, became the world's best-known scientist: the woman whose work would save mankind from the scourge of cancer.

Of course it was not that simple. But with surgery and chemotherapy, ionizing radiation is still one of the principal methods of treating cancer, and the range of sources available to the radiotherapist is continually increasing. Implants of radioactive materials, similar to the radium needles, are used for some cancers. But for many years now the bulk of treatment has been given with a beam of X-rays or gamma rays from one of the big machines.

Implants

Better understanding of the effects of radiation on tissues means that doctors now know much more accurately what dose of radiation they should give to a particular tumour in a particular place. Radium needles, whose output is difficult to control, have been abandoned in favour of irridium wires and small cylinders of radioactive caesium, which are in any case much safer to handle than radium. The activity from these implants will only travel from about 1 mm to, at most, a couple of centimetres, so they need to be implanted as close as possible to the tumour. The wires can actually be inserted into the tumour as the radium needles were. Caesium comes in larger pieces, and is normally used to treat cancers in a body cavity, like the uterus, for instance. This sort of implant may be left in position for anything between 24 hours and 7 days, and then removed. Other implants, like minute grains of radioactive gold, which are sometimes injected into glands in the neck, can be left permanently. They have a half-life of only 2.7 days (compared with 37 years for caesium) and once they have lost the bulk of their activity the grains will have no further effect.

Injections

Another way of 'implanting' a radioactive source into a particular part of the body is to inject it into the bloodstream and leave it to find its own way. Radioactive iodine is an example. Any iodine in the body is avidly taken up by the thyroid gland, because iodine is incorporated into thyroxine, a thyroid hormone. A radioactive isotope of iodine behaves in the same way, so this is often how overactive thyroid glands are treated. Similarly a radioactive isotope of phosphorus can be used in treating a cancer of the red blood cells, because phosphorus is taken up by the cells in the bone marrow which are involved in making red blood cells. Research is going on in many centres now to see whether this guiding of radioactive isotopes to a particular destination can be taken a step further, by attaching the isotopes to monoclonal antibodies which are designed to home in on a cancer target.

Big machines

The power and dose of X-rays given for treatment is enormously different from the amount received by a person 'having an X-ray done'. A diagnostic X-ray machine would have a power of about 100 keV (1000 electron-volts) and one exposure would last for less than a second. The dose for, say, a chest X-ray is of the order of 1/1000 of a rad, or in more modern parlance, .00001 Gray. A tumour might well be given a dose from a 10 meV (million electron-volts) machine of 60 Gray, 6 million times as much.

Normally treatment given in the form of a beam of radiation from one of the big machines will be with either X- or gamma rays. They are more or less interchangeable, being the same thing, but from different sources. Whereas the X-rays are produced electrically, gamma rays are emitted by a radioactive substance.

Cobalt bombs: A 'cobalt bomb', containing cobalt 60, is the commonest source of gamma radiation. The cobalt is totally enclosed in a bulky treatment head which absorbs the radiation when the machine is not in use. To use the beam, either the cobalt is moved into line with the aperture or a shutter is opened. Cobalt 60 has a half-life of a little over five years, which means that the intensity of radiation is halved in that

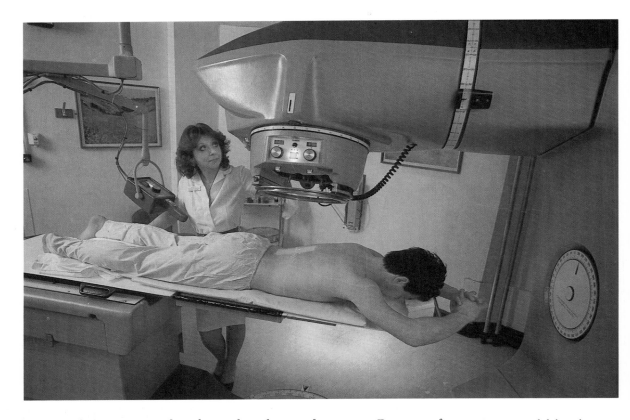

time, so the source needs to be replaced every few years. But apart from that, a cobalt 60 source is easier to operate and maintain than a high-energy X-ray source. However, whereas the cobalt unit produces gamma rays at 1 meV, the bottom of the high-energy range, linear accelerators can go much higher.

Less powerful than the linear accelerator, a cobalt source is used to treat more localised disease, like the painful secondary tumours that can occur in bone

Linear accelerators: Within limits, the higher the energy of the X-rays the deeper they penetrate, and the greater the dose at the target compared with the dose at the skin. That is why linear accelerators are the most useful X-ray sources for radiation therapy. A typical linear accelerator is a long copper tube, inside which a radio-frequency wave is travelling in an electric field. Electrons from an electron gun are injected into the beginning of this wave guide, and any that arrive immediately in front of the negative field will stay there and be pushed along, rather like a surf rider on the crest of a wave. The electrons that miss that part of the wave will come in on the next one. The inside surface of the tube is structured so that the electrons are carried faster and faster, emerging from the tube at very nearly the speed of light, and in the treatment head they collide with a target, usually of tungsten, which emits very high-voltage X-rays. Occasionally the tungsten target is removed and the electrons themselves are used in treatment, particularly in skin cancers, because a beam of electrons has the advantage that it is effective to a certain depth, and then stops dead.

The power of linear accelerators varies. A typical one used in a British hospital would have a power of about 8 or 10 meV. (Curiously enough the appropriate energy of machine adopted by a country depends on the average size of its people. In Japan they go for 6–8 meV. Whether that will change with the arrival in that country of MacDonald's hamburgers is a question.) There are much bigger, more powerful machines, 20–25, even 35 meV, but they tend to be used more for treatments like whole body irradiation, when the patient has to be at a much greater distance from the machine, than when the target is a tumour.

Aiming the big machines

Unfortunately there is no form of radiation that damages only cancer cells; but the difference between cancer and normal tissue gives the normal cells some advantage. A normal adult cell will only divide when it is necessary for a new cell to be made to replace an old one that has died. In cancer this control mechanism breaks down, and a cancer cell carries on reproducing all the time regardless of whether any replacement is necessary. This means that at any one time a much larger proportion of the cancer cells are in the course of division, or preparing for division, than is usually the case among the surrounding normal tissue. This helps the radiotherapist, because although cells can be

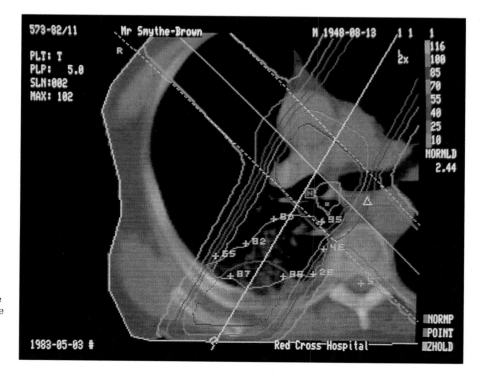

Computer calculation of the radiation dose that would be received by various organs as a result of two intersecting beams of X-rays.

damaged by radiation at any time, they appear to be much more vulnerable when they are preparing to divide or actually doing so. In addition, because the normal cells have this ability to respond in a controlled way to replace lost cells, they appear to repair the damage caused by the radiation much more effectively than the cancer does.

In the early days of radiation therapy those undergoing treatment did suffer very badly from damage to normal tissues, particularly burning of the skin. This led the radiotherapists to try breaking up the dose into a number of separate sessions. There was no carefully devised rationale for this, but it worked, and effects on the skin were less severe. A course of radiotherapy now is normally spread out over four to six weeks, with treatments daily or three times a week. This gives normal tissue a chance to recover between sessions.

The most important factor of all, however, is the geometry: making sure that the cancer receives a higher dose of radiation than the normal tissue surrounding it. This is easy if the cancer is in the skin or very near the surface, but what if it is a deep cancer, for example in the bladder? Depending on its source, the beam of radiation is at its most powerful at or a little below the skin. By the time it reaches the bladder it may even be as low as 40-60 per cent of its original power. So it appears inevitable that the intervening tissue must receive a higher dose than the tumour. To overcome this, the treatment is planned in what might be called, a 'searchlight pattern'. Searchlight beams from many different directions converge on the target, the enemy plane. So the plane receives a 'dose' which is the sum of all the beams. The space through which each beam passes is illuminated by one source. Of course, the radiotherapy machine has only one source, so the beams are applied one after the other rather than at the same time, but the effect is similar.

The vulnerability to radiation damage of different types of healthy tissue varies a great deal. Normal cells of the lining of the gut and lung, for instance, are very much more likely to be damaged than are those of the kidney and liver, so this also enters the calculations when a regime of radiation therapy is being planned.

The factor that sets the upper limit on the dose of radiation, wherever on the body the tumour may be, is usually the effect on one type of cell; lymphocytes, the white blood cells from which most of the components of the immune system are made, are exceptionally vulnerable to radiation damage. For some reason the lymphocytes are not only affected in the same way as other cells; they also appear somehow to be induced to destroy themselves. This is always a problem, but particularly so when a large area is being treated. Since the lymphocytes are components of blood, and continuously on the move, it is likely that a high proportion of the total population will have passed under the beam at some time during the treatment. So throughout a course of radiation treatments a continuous check is kept on the white cell count, and if it drops too low the treatment has to be temporally suspended.

Effects on the cell

Although the effect of radiation on cells is not completely understood, there is no doubt that the main effect is on the nucleus. Ionizing radiation is able to dislodge an electron from any atom it collides with. When it collides with part of the DNA in the nucleus then it can cause a change or break. If the damage is not repaired then it may be serious enough to kill the cell outright. Alternatively the cell may simply lose its ability to reproduce.

One fact about radiation that has limited its effectiveness, and is possibly the reason why so many treated tumours tend to regrow, is the oxygen effect; cells are much less vulnerable to radiation damage if they are short of oxygen. A tumour usually manages to grab more than its fair share of any available oxygen so its outer layers are well oxygenated, but when it is large there may be cells at its centre that are very poorly supplied, and these are the ones that may survive.

When a collision happens and an electron is knocked off, a number of things can happen:

- the electron may fall back again to repair the damage;
- the atom from which the electron was dislodged may react immediately with a neighbouring atom that has also been ionized;
- the electron may be trapped by a roaming oxygen atom leaving the damaged atom in a highly reactive state.

Free oxygen has a powerful attraction for loose electrons, so if there is plenty of oxygen around the last possibility is a likely one and the cell will be killed. When oxygen is short there is much more chance that the first alternative will result, and so the cell will survive and provide a focus from which the tumour can grow again.

If the oxygen effect can be overcome the outcome of radiotherapy may be significantly improved. One possibility is to try to flood the tissues, including the cancer, with oxygen. In a number of trials patients have been given their treatments while lying in oxygen chambers pumped up to three times the normal atmospheric pressure, but the results were disappointing. Although it works in experimental tumours in animals, in the majority of humans it seems to make very little difference. And it complicates the procedure enormously, so for the time being at least the idea has been abandoned.

The opposite approach, starving the normal tissues of oxygen, has also been unsuccessful. The idea was to stop the flow of blood to the area of the tumour by applying a tourniquet, so obviously it was only practicable on a tumour in a place like a leg or arm. When a resource like oxygen is scarce a tumour is likely to be more successful in competition for it than normal tissue, so the oxygen shortage would appear in the surrounding tissue before affecting the tumour. Thus reducing blood flow should make the normal cells less vulnerable without affecting the cancer cells. It should, but in a number of trials it was ineffective, so that, too, has been abandoned.

Radiosensitizers

There are a number of drugs that can perform the role the oxygen plays in maximizing radiation damage. Chemicals with an affinity for electrons can mop them up in the same way as the oxygen does. Unfortunately no drug has yet been found that can be given in sufficient quantities to increase the 'oxygen effect' significantly without serious side effects. However, scientists working on one drug (a substance normally used to treat some types of infection) have now succeeded in producing a less toxic version which they hope may be suitable. Meanwhile there is another approach.

Fast neutrons

When the British physicist James Chadwick first discovered neutrons in 1939 he suggested that they might be helpful in treating cancer, and a beam of fast neutrons should be much less influenced by the oxygen effect. The neutrons themselves do not cause ionization damage. What they do is collide with atoms, and the collisions release a variety of ionizing particles, all of which act in the immediate vicinity of the collision. Because so much damage is being caused in one place at one time there is very little chance of electrons being recaptured to repair the damage.

The most effective way of producing fast neutrons is with a cyclotron. A stream of very pure hydrogen is passed over an electric arc which knocks off the electrons. The resulting protons are then fed into the centre of a vacuum chamber, where they are held in a magnetic field while they are accelerated round and round a flat spiral orbit by an

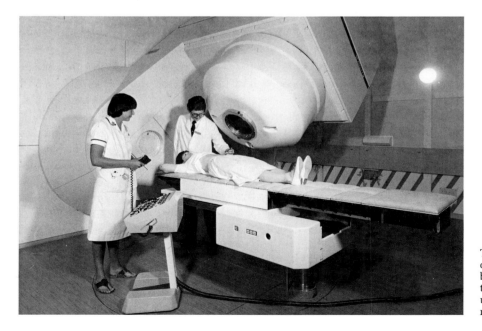

The massive treatment head of a cyclotron which uses a beam of fast neutrons to treat cancers that are unaffected by other types of radiotherapy

alternating current. At the end of their spiral path, when the particles are travelling at one third of the speed of light, they are deflected out along a tube, where they are still held by a series of magnets which can steer them around corners and into the treatment head. This is the part of the machine that can be manoeuvred into position over a patient, and inside it the stream of high energy protons collides with a target of beryllium, producing a shower of protons, electrons and neutrons. The protons and electrons, being charged, are captured almost immediately by the surrounding material in the treatment head, leaving a beam of high energy neutrons: which was the object of the exercise.

Until recently there have been only a handful of low-powered cyclotrons at the disposal of hospitals, and so the only trials of neutron beam therapy have been on tumours in accessible places like the head and neck. However, since the beginning of the 1980s a few cyclotrons of comparable power to the big linear accelerators have been built in hospitals, and with these it will be possible to try out the effects on a much greater range of tumours.

Future prospects
As well as providing neutrons, cyclotrons are able to produce a vast range of radioactive isotopes which are used both in implants and to assist in diagnosis of disease (page 41). They also give radiotherapists a chance to try out the possibilities of other types of subatomic particle. By simply removing the beryllium target the proton beam itself can be used to treat some types of cancer; by varying the energy of the beam it is possible to arrange that the particles are at their most damaging precisely when they reach the tumour. Pi-mesons, another form of subatomic particle, have much the same ability to travel harmlessly, then after a certain distance become unstable and disintegrate explosively. They are being used in trials on brain tumours.

Another quite different part of the electromagnetic spectrum - in fact the opposite end - is already believed by many people to be able to help the healing of broken bones. Now it is also being used experimentally to fight cancer. Radio-frequency waves do not cause ionization, but the idea is to focus the waves on to a tumour and heat it to a temperature of 5°C above normal. This has been shown to stop tumours growing, but whether it will prove better than other more established treatments is still being investigated. The same principle of overheating the area of the tumour is also being followed by other doctors, but using ultrasound rather than radio waves to produce the temperature rise.

At the same time as work is going on with the newer particles and radio and ultrasound, a better understanding of the physics of radiation and its biological effects is being built up. This should lead to more precise ways of tailoring the treatment to each individual tumour, so that the greatest benefit can be achieved with the lowest possible level of unwanted side effects.

CHAPTER SEVEN

Spare Parts

In running a spares service for human beings the medical profession has two sources of supply: one is industry – engineering, chemical, electronic; the other is nature – parts of animals or humans, dead or alive. Each type of spare part has its advantages and disadvantages. For the more complicated components nature beats industry hands down on fitness for purpose and micro-miniaturization, and the parts are much cheaper; but there are problems of rejection, and of course supply does not always match demand. Industry often provides rather good structural spare parts, their shelf life is better than the natural variety and, laying aside cost, they can be provided to order or made to measure. However, man-made spares of functional parts are nearly always only partial substitutes, and they are normally bulky and inconvenient.

Structural members

From the cosmetic point of view, prosthetic limbs have come a long way since the days of Long John Silver and Captain Hook. Artificial legs and arms are designed now to look as much as possible like the real thing, bearing in mind that they have to be able to function. A satisfactory artificial leg is much easier to achieve than an artificial arm because the range of movement required is so much simpler, and people become amazingly adept at walking, and even climbing, with artificial legs. A replacement for an arm may not need to be as strong as a leg, but it requires a much greater range of movement; and a satisfactory artificial arm would need a hand that could demonstrate some strength and a great deal of dexterity.

In recent years considerable progress has been made in creating artificial limbs that respond to some degree to the intentions in the mind of the owner. When we decide to move an arm our brains send an electric signal down the relevant nerves. These are passed on to the muscle fibres, and an electric current is produced as the muscle fibres are stimulated. The best artificial arm at the moment, the myoelectric limb, operates by picking up signals from any muscle fibres the person wearing the arm has remaining. These signals are relayed to small motors which operate about six movements, opening and closing the hand, bending and straightening the elbow, and turning the wrist. The development of these limbs is an impressive achievement, but apart from the fact that this is a limited range compared with a normal arm, they can only be used by people who still have a fair amount of their original arm.

A much greater range might be achieved if the arm could be switched directly by the signals in the nerves that control the muscle fibres. But that is much more difficult; whereas muscle signals can be picked up on the surface of the skin, electrodes to pick up the much weaker nerve signals would need to be implanted surgically, and to avoid wires passing through the skin (always carrying a danger of infection), any signals would have to be transmitted to the arm by radio. People

Knee joint specially designed to be fixed without use of cement

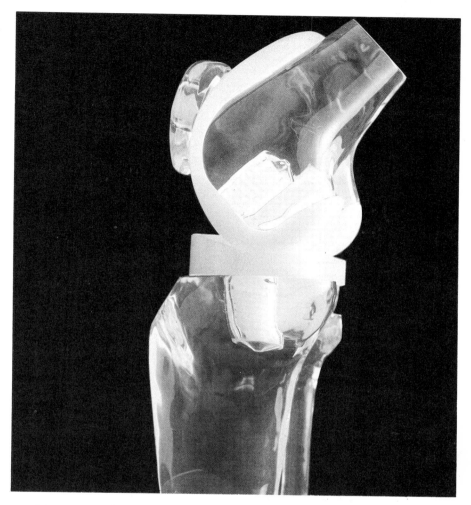

working on such control mechanisms are convinced that this can be done, and tests in animals have shown that it is possible to pick up the signals coming down a nerve to control the movement of a limb. These still have to be analysed, to see whether it is possible to pick out signal patterns and harness them to motors, to provide a greater range of movement than is available in the arms operated by muscle signals.

Joint replacements

Orthopaedic surgeons are not the only people who would agree that probably one of the most successful operations the world has ever known is the total hip replacement. Although shoulders, elbows, ankles, knuckles, wrists and toes are also possible, by far the most commonly replaced joint is the hip (half a million every year throughout the world), followed by the knee. These are the main weight-bearing joints, and so they take the greatest punishment. The average person in walking or moving about generally puts pressure on his hip and knee joints about two million times a year, and the loading is as a rule about twice bodyweight: in really athletic activity the load on a knee can be more than 20 times the weight. When they do wear out it is usually for one of two reasons: either rheumatoid arthritis, when many of the joints become red and inflamed and the immune system attacks the joint lining; or because of osteoarthritis in which pain and inflammation are the result of wear and tear on the joint rather than being the original cause. This type of wear is often the long-term result of a slight physical deformity, and this kind of damage is five times as common as rheumatoid arthritis, affecting about like five million people in Britain alone.

The operation to replace a damaged hip is more common than that for the knee for two reasons. One is the design of the joints – it is easier to produce a stable ball-and-socket joint like the hip, and it is firmly held by muscles. The knee is more like a hinge and a stable substitute has proved much more difficult to achieve. The second reason is that a damaged knee is much easier to endure than a damaged hip. There are just as many people suffering painful knees, but they are only painful part of the time. When the owner of a damaged knee is sitting or lying down the knee stops hurting.

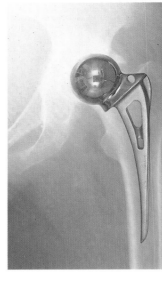

X-ray of a hip replacement

In the normal joint the two bones, hip and thigh, or thigh and shin, are separated by a thick layer of cartilage, a gristly substance which is very tough. But it is also porous, and its surface contains a fluid which squeezes out of it to lubricate the joint as it moves. Cartilage contains no nerves, so the smooth movement of a normal joint even under loading is painless. In arthritis the cartilage wears away, or tears or cracks, the bone is damaged and begins to grow abnormally at the edges, producing a misshapen, knobbly joint which moves jerkily, sticks and is acutely painful. In the hip, because of the ball-and-socket shape of the joint and the large powerful muscles holding it in position, the two surfaces are always in contact, so even at rest a movement of the hip joint can be painful. In the knee, the two surfaces can separate slightly when the joint is not bearing weight, so movement causes little or no pain.

The normal hip is a ball and socket, and so is the replacement joint. The ball part is mounted on a shaft which is driven deep into the marrow cavity at the top of the thighbone, or femur. The socket fits into a hollowed-out space in the hipbone. When joint replacement operations began nobody was sure how well they would stand up to wear, so they tended only to be done for elderly patients who were unlikely to need their new joints for very many years; and indeed the surface of the hip socket of the earliest joints did wear out. To reduce friction to a minimum these sockets were lined with PTFE (the non-stick material used in frying pans), and tiny particles of this wore away causing reaction in the joints. Now the socket part of the joint is made of very strong dense solid plastic, and the ball of metal, usually either titanium alloy, stainless steel or an alloy of cobalt-chrome-molybdenum.

Because joint replacement operations are so successful, younger and younger people are asking for them, which means that the demand made on the replacement joints is growing. The amount of stress that a joint will suffer in the 20 years' expectation of life of a 50-year-old is a great deal less than in the life ahead of an energetic man of 30. So the weak points are being revealed, and the weakest point is the cement that holds the pieces in position.

The cement is not used as glue, more as a filler to pack the space round both halves of the new joint where they fit into the top of the thighbone and into the hipbone. The metal joint is, as a rule, less flexible than the bone, so the stress of wear is particularly severe at the junction of cement with bone. Not only that, but the bone is living material and at least in the early days a sort of immune reaction sometimes began at the bone–cement interface. During this reaction the surface of the bone was damaged, and the bond broke down. New cements have been developed which reduce this problem, but many surgeons believe that the best solution is wherever possible to abandon the cement.

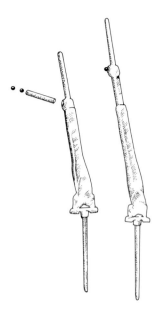

BELOW Design for an artificial thighbone that 'grows' with a growing child

Knee joint replacements that rely entirely on plastic plugs to hold them in place have been available for some years. Holes are drilled in the bone ends, and the plugs are hammered in. They have a series of flanges, rather like a screw thread but non-continuous, and the bone regrows in between the flanges of the plugs to grip the joint components firmly. The glueless version of the hip joint is still only at an experimental stage. One solution for the thighbone component is to make it with a triangular cross-section shaft which is driven into the marrow cavity of the bone and wedged into position with bone grafts. For the cup component, which fits into the hipbone, the idea is to mount the plastic cup into a metal holder which is screwed into a threaded socket cut into the bone. The metal of both parts is titanium, because it appears that bone will grow more closely to titanium than any other metal, and the idea is that the growing bone will form itself to grip the metal tightly. Another solution for the metal component has been simply to roughen the surface of the shaft, leaving small irregularities into which tiny fingers of bone can grow and knit the bond tightly.

As long as the shaft of the joint is made of metal it is likely to be more rigid than the growing bone, and that creates stresses, so attempts are being made to fashion this component out of newer materials. One idea is to make a composite part, with the fixing shaft made of carbon fibre-reinforced epoxy resin, and the ball made of a ceramic material. The ceramic is very smooth, creating little friction, and one extra advantage is that whereas metal becomes rougher as it wears, the effect of wear on a ceramic material is to make it smoother and glassier.

Scaffolding

There are some diseases like cancer that eat away steadily at bones. Until recently, the only solution has been to amputate the limb, but artificial bone and joint replacements can now make that unnecessary for a few people at least. The implants can replace a large part of the bone of a limb – from the hip to the shinbone, for example – and they are made to measure out of metals or plastics, usually a combination of both. Their big advantage over an artificial limb is that all the nervous and muscle control apparatus may be saved, so the limb can work more or less normally – particularly important in the arm. A scheme has even been developed to make these implants suitable for children, because the bone replacement can be made to grow, if not gradually as the living child, at least in ball bearing-sized steps. A telescopic 'bone' consists of a metal sleeve with a piston inside it. The length of the 'bone' is extended by pushing the piston further and further out of the sleeve, and it is fixed in this extended position by injecting a series of tungsten-carbide ball bearings into the sleeve through a small incision in the skin.

As well as the artificial joint replacements, there have been some attempts at transplantation of bones and joints from dead donors, but they are already less convenient than the artificial kind, and the latter are improving all the time. Some components, like terylene and carbon fibre ligaments, are actually stronger than the natural ones.

Skin

There is no artificial skin at the moment that can permanently take the place of the natural kind. When the various substitutes are used, either the natural skin repairs itself underneath or in the end a graft is needed. Patches can now be grown from a few of a person's own skin cells, and one alternative being tried involves laying over the wound a scaffolding of fibres of collagen, perhaps taken from an animal, and sowing this scaffolding with a few of the person's own skin cells which might grow to fill the spaces between the fibres. With both techniques the resulting skin would not be quite the same as normal skin, having no sweat glands or hair follicles.

Pumps, pipes and processing plant

Bionic man is nowhere near being a possibility. Although there are good replacements for joints and bones, and some excellent small components, when it comes to working organs of the human body good bionic spares are very much a thing of the future.

The heart

The simplest working organ of the human body is probably the heart. It is, after all, just a pump, although a most elegantly designed one. De-oxygenated venous blood enters the heart through the right atrium and passes through a one-way valve to the right ventricle, from which it is pumped under fairly low pressure into the lungs, where it is re-oxygenated. It then returns to the heart via the left atrium, and through another one-way valve it enters the left ventricle from which it is

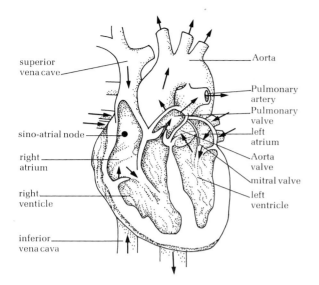

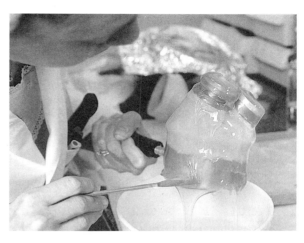

ABOVE LEFT The heart with its major blood vessels
ABOVE RIGHT The Jarvik artificial heart, the first artificial heart designed to be a permanent replacement

pumped at higher pressure round the body. So the heart pump has to be able to coordinate a double pumping action at different pressures. The normal human heart can also respond to hormonal and electrical signals telling it to speed up or slow down or to pump more or less strongly. Normal resting heart rate is about 70 beats a minute, but when an athlete runs a race, when his muscles make very much increased demands on the oxygen from his blood, his heart rate responds by speeding up to as much as 200 beats a minute. In the opposite direction, it is said that Eastern mystics can slow their bodies down by profound relaxation so that their heart rate drops to less than 10 a minute.

So an artificial heart needs a mechanism robust enough to perform a double pumping action 40 million times a year, a power supply capable of providing the energy for those 40 million heartbeats, and a control mechanism to vary the output, preferably automatically.

Two different basic types of artificial heart have so far been put into human beings. The first was in 1969 and was implanted by Denton Cooley, the famous Texan heart surgeon. It was designed to be simply a temporary replacement for the patient's failing heart, to be removed as soon as a suitably matched donor heart became available for a transplant, and there are many people who think that this is likely to be the only sensible kind of use for artificial hearts.

A man-made heart that was not designed to be only a temporary stopgap was fitted into the chest of Dr Barney Clark, a retired dentist, by a team in Salt Lake City, Utah, in 1982. It consisted of two plastic spheres each containing a diaphragm which was driven up and down by compressed air to suck in the blood and push it out again. To fit the device, most of Dr Clark's own heart was cut away, and the replacement was joined on to the remnants of the atria by dacron cuffs. The blood entered the pumping chambers of the heart through two valves and was driven out via large dacron tubes into the pulmonary artery and aorta.

Barney Clark lived with his artificial heart for nearly four months.

Because the doctors were worried that the mechanical action of the heart might damage the blood and lead to clotting, he was given large doses of anticoagulant drugs. These drugs may have been partly responsible for the damage to his other organs which ultimately led to his death, and it seems that they may have over-estimated the likelihood of clotting. They also think the new heart work too hard for his other organs which were already wasted after his long illness.

Since Dr Clark's death there has been a great deal of controversy about whether any more of these operations should be carried out until much more development work has been done on the heart. Nevertheless there have been a few further implants, using some of the lessons learned from the first case. The surgeons concerned feel that there is a lot they can learn from using the existing model, but they plan only to use one when a natural transplant, which has a much better chance of success, and offers an immeasurably better quality of life, is out of the question.

The real problem that has to be overcome is the power source. Barney Clark's heart was driven with compressed air, and the apparatus to supply this was mounted on a trolley weighing 170 kg (375 lb). Wherever he went the trolley went with him. The power pack has now been reduced to the size of a briefcase, but it lasts for only three or four hours and then needs recharging, so the problem is still far from being solved. It is generally agreed that artificial hearts will never be anything other than experimental until a really small and reliable power source, so small and reliable that it can be implanted inside the body, is available. The likeliest contenders as sources of power are nuclear energy or some kind of electro-chemical process.

An acceptable artificial heart may not be developed until the twenty-first century, but individual components are available off the shelf now. When valves fail they can be replaced either with natural ones or with a mechanical equivalent. The biological valves come sometimes from humans and sometimes from animals such as pigs. They can be removed and sterilized with antibiotics or other chemicals, and they can even be freeze-dried. As an alternative to the real thing they may be built up out of other human tissue. Unlike whole organs, valves do not create rejection problems, so there is no need for tissue compatibility testing, and those designed for the job by nature do it very well. They do have one disadvantage compared with the mechanical kind: no one is quite sure how long they will last. Many people who have had replacement valves in the past, particularly those built up from human tissue, are now coming into hospital for the second time round, and it seems that a reasonable expectation for the life of such a valve may not be much more than ten years. Mechanical valves, on the other hand, should last for as long as their owners have need of them, although one type did have to be withdrawn because it suffered from metal fatigue. One disadvantage of mechanical valves is that because they contain foreign materials the blood can stick to them, causing clotting, so the wearer

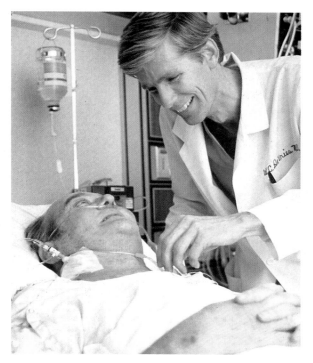

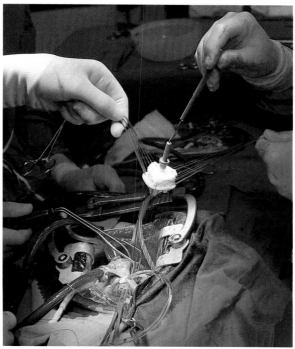

will probably need to take some kind of anticoagulant drug for the rest of his life. Also many of the artificial valves are hydrodynamically different from the natural kind, and any turbulence they create may do some damage to red cells. Nevertheless, many people live very happily with them.

Failure of heart valves is often the long-term result of rheumatic heart disease, and as that has become much less common in the developed world, so too should the need for valve replacement. Failure of the coronary arteries, however, which keep the heart muscle supplied with blood, is becoming all too common, and they also can be replaced, or usually bypassed, either with natural or artificial blood vessels. The natural kind are in fact not arteries but veins, and come from the individual's own legs where nature has provided more than enough veins to cope with the returning blood. Developing satisfactory substitutes for these smaller blood vessels has proved much more difficult than might be expected. Dacron or other synthetic large vessels have been available for years, and give excellent service as replacements for vessels such as the aorta, but small vessels have been a problem because they tend to become blocked. However smooth and glassy the inside surface of a plastic tube, the blood still manages to stick to it, clots may form and possibly break off and cause a total blockage. The cells of the inner walls of living arteries produce a chemical called prostacyclin which is specifically designed to stop this happening. The developers of the latest design of artificial vessels have abandoned any attempt to make the inner surfaces smooth; instead they have deliberately made them rough inside, and the cells seep in among the fibres and lay down a natural surface to which the flowing blood does not stick.

Pacemakers

The other main component of the heart that can be replaced now is the control mechanism. Unlike other muscles, the heart is at least partly independent of the brain in command of its own nervous signals. The signal which triggers each heartbeat begins at the top of the right atrium, at a point called the sino-atrial node (SA node) and travels across the heart through specially adapted tissue, in such a way that the filling and pumping action is correctly coordinated. If this goes wrong either the heart can slow down dangerously or even stop altogether, or it can speed up or become hopelessly irregular. When that begins to happen the answer may well be an electric pacemaker; more than half a million have been fitted.

A permanent pacemaker consists of one or two wires leading to the heart from a matchbox-sized control box implanted just below the skin – normally on the chest. The matchbox contains a pulse generator, powered by a lithium battery which has a life of up to 15 years, and usually a microprocessor. In the early days the fitting of a pacemaker involved a major operation, opening the chest and attaching the wire to the outside of the ventricles. Now the wires are fed into the heart through a vein, and they operate from inside the heart muscle. If the problem is not that the conduction of signals through the heart is faulty, but that the natural pacemaker, the SA node, has broken down, then the wire normally goes to the atrium. But often the problem is with the passage of signals within the heart, and then the pacemaker wire leads to the ventricles, because that is the really the crucial pumping part. Pacemakers are usually arranged so that they are inactive when the heart is beating normally of its own accord, only switching into action when the natural beat fails. In the early days they were simply set at about 70 beats per minute and were not variable, except by an operation to gain access to the mechanism. Most modern pacemakers can have their pulse-generating controls changed by radio signals, and many have automatically variable controls built in.

The first models that could increase their rate automatically when the body demanded extra oxygen would only work properly in people whose sino-atrial nodes were producing proper pulses, and who needed their pacemakers because the transmission of the signals through the heart had broken down. They worked by picking up the signal from the SA node with one wire and carrying it up to the pacemaker control where it was amplified and sent back down to trigger the ventricle: so if the SA node speeded up so did the signal to the ventricle, and therefore the heart's pumping action. It was not until 1981 that the pacemaker users who had faulty signals from the SA node (about half of all the users) could have a model that responded to their body's oxygen demand. This became possible when it was discovered that the hormones like adrenalin that tell the SA node how frequently to fire also have a direct effect on the heart muscle cells, making them

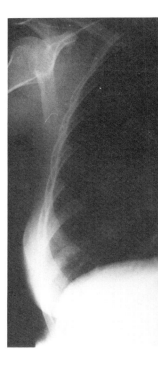

A heart pacemaker in position with wire leading to the pumping chamber

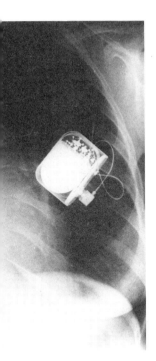

recover more quickly after conducting impulses. So a pacemaker has been developed that senses how fast the muscle cells are responding to its signal. The faster the response the more adrenalin must be around, and therefore the faster the pacemaker should fire.

Another method of controlling pacemakers which is still under development would use a bio-sensor, a chip that is able to detect the presence of chemicals. It consists of an outer layer of the material that responds to the chemical, and an inner layer of electronic chip which produces the signal to send to the processor, in this case the pacemaker, telling it to speed up or slow down as necessary. There is no obvious reason why such a chip should not be developed to sense the presence of adrenalin, oxygen, hydrogen, glucose, etc., and research into such systems is in progress at the moment.

Some of the most recently developed pacemakers even keep a record of their own activity and can transmit this to a recorder which the doctor can examine when there is trouble or when the patient comes in for a regular check. In fact, often there is no need for the patient to visit the hospital for this check, since the record can be 'phoned in' over an ordinary telephone line.

Pacemakers can cope with many types of slow or irregular heartbeat, and some can even stop the condition known as ventricular tachycardia, when the heart beats so fast that the ventricles are unable to fill with blood, although this calls for a special pacemaker programmed to recognize an impending attack and break the rhythm with a special pattern of signals. But no pacemaker is able to handle the worst case, the heart going into fibrillation, when the beat is not much more than a random twitching, and the heart is said to resemble a bag of worms. The usual pacemaker signal is not strong enough to correct these dangerous conditions; the defibrillator, which is part of the cardiac resuscitation equipment, delivers a real electrical kick to the heart to knock it back into rhythm. An implantable defibrillator has now been developed and is being tried out in a number of centres. It is very much like the pacemaker, but with one electrode inside the heart and one attached to the outside, and a control box and batteries under the skin, but the defibrillator delivers a pulse of 25 joules, a million times the current of the normal pacemaker. Like the pacemaker it can be programmed to recognize fibrillation and automatically deliver a shock to deal with it.

The lungs

Nobody has yet developed anything in the way of implantable lungs, but their work can be done outside the body. Most open heart operations are performed with the work of the patient's lungs and heart taken over by a machine. In the traditional heart–lung machine (if a life of 25 years can be called a tradition) the blood is piped out of the body into a flask where oxygen is bubbled through it. This allows the blood to pick up oxygen and release carbon dioxide. This works satisfactorily for a short time, but the bumping and bubbling can damage some of the red cells, and after some hours the damage becomes permanent. So when the lungs need resting for longer periods a different system is used. This is the membrane oxygenator, which consists of a sandwich of membranes which are semi-permeable: gas can penetrate, blood cannot. It is really just like a normal lung, but where in the lungs the gas is in the alveoli and blood in minute capillaries, separated by the walls of the vessels, in the oxygenator the blood and gas are in layers separated by the membranes. Because of the difference in partial pressures of the gases in the two layers, the oxygen diffuses into the blood and the CO_2 diffuses out. The artificial lung allows the gases to be exchanged very efficiently. It needs to, because there are only a few square metres of membrane, whereas the 300 million alveoli in the lungs provide an area something like the size of a tennis court.

Blood

Blood is comparatively easy to transplant, and because live donors can be used (in Britain for the price of a cup of tea and a biscuit), supply and demand are in reasonable equilibrium. However, blood for transfusion does have to be correctly matched and can go out of date, so there are some advantages in the artificial kind that has been developed. It is not a complete substitute, but carries out just one of blood's many functions, the transport of oxygen. In blood most of the oxygen is carried on the haemoglobin molecule with which the red cells are packed. The haemoglobin does not grip the oxygen tightly; it has been described as 'more of a handshake', so it is easily released to fuel the various cells of the body on demand. Instead of haemoglobin, the artificial blood contains molecules of fluorocarbon, which perform the same function, picking up oxygen in the lungs and releasing it to the oxygen-hungry tissues. The artificial blood is seen only as a standby for real blood in all except one situation. Following the type of stroke that is due to a blocked artery in the brain there is an urgent need to get oxygen through to the tissues. The fluorocarbon molecule is only one-hundredth the size of a red cell and there may sometimes be just enough space in the blocked artery to allow the fluorocarbon molecules to pass where the haemoglobin cannot.

Kidneys

If the job of the lung is to correct the gases in the blood, it is the job of the kidneys and liver to correct pretty well everthing else. The liver's role is so complicated that it is difficult to imagine how any artificial organ could take over more than a minute part of it. The kidney machine, on the other hand, can keep a person alive for many years. It was the first artificial organ to be produced.

In the kidney the blood passes through a structure in which water, salts, virtually everything except the cells and large proteins, are re-

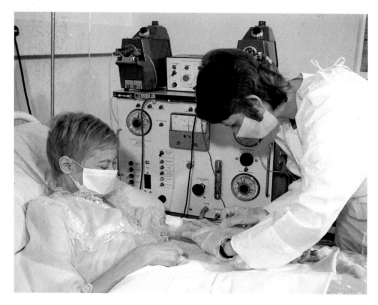

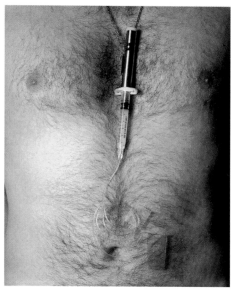

ABOVE LEFT Renal dialysis in hospital. The kidney was the first organ to be replaced by a machine

ABOVE RIGHT The average patient using this insulin pump would not have to refill for about four days

moved. The resulting fluid then passes into a system where cells reclaim all the useful bits, like most of the water, salts and nutrients, and feed them back into the bloodstream. Some of the water, and the unwanted waste materials like urea, are eliminated as urine. The kidney is able to correct the balance of many of the constituents of the blood, re-absorbing only the required amount of substances like salts, sugar and water, and it can even change the balance on instructions from hormones. It also makes a number of hormones itself.

The artificial kidney is a less subtle organ. It is much less able to distinguish between wanted and unwanted substances than the real kidney, and of course it cannot make its own hormones, or vary its action on instructions from other hormones; but it can remove from the blood some of the waste products which if they remained would mean certain death. In an artificial kidney the blood is removed from the body and passes over a semi-permeable membrane, made of cellophane. On the other side is a fluid which causes the unwanted waste constituents to filter across the membrane by diffusion, and the cleaned blood is then returned to the body. A large area of membrane is needed, with plenty of fluid, so the patient is tied to a bulky apparatus for three 5–6 hour sessions a week: a far cry from the 140 gm (5 oz) of natural kidney.

In some ways the process known as CAPD (continuous ambulatory peritoneal dialysis) is closer to the normal kidney, because it does not involve being tied to a machine. This uses the peritoneum, the largest membrane in the body, as its semi-permeable membrane for the diffusion process, and it is happening all the time. The peritoneal cavity, which surrounds the intestines and other organs of the abdomen, is filled with dialysing fluid from a bag the person wears round his waist, via a tube which is left permanently in place. Impurities from the blood filter across the peritoneum which surrounds the whole of this cavity, into the fluid, which is allowed to drain back into its bag at the end of 6–8 hours, and the process begins all over again. The main danger of this is that it can cause infection, and of course it is still a very partial substitute. The best treatment for kidney failure at the moment is undoubtedly a transplant.

Pancreas

Many organs of our bodies are known by their failures rather than their successes, so the one thing we all know about the pancreas is that it produces insulin, and that in diabetes that insulin production fails. Without insulin the body is unable to use glucose from sugar and other carbohydrates in the diet, and so it builds up to dangerous levels in the blood and the cells are starved. The pancreas does much more than make insulin, but when people talk about an artificial pancreas they mean a mechanism that will deliver insulin to the blood at a rate that will control blood glucose. There have been forecasts that an implantable artificial pancreas that can perform this task will be produced in 1985. If it is, it will need (a) a sensor to monitor the blood glucose, (b) a processor to convert this reading into an estimate of the dose of insulin that is needed, (c) a method of releasing insulin and (d) a reservoir to hold a long-term supply of the hormone.

(a) It is possible that the sensor may be a bio-chip. The outer layer of this bio-chip would contain an enzyme capable of breaking down glucose into simpler components, producing a small electric current which could be detected by the chip. An alternative method would use a platinum catalyst to break down the glucose.

(b) The microcomputer could be programmed with all the information to enable it to calculate how much, if any, insulin it should deliver, and at what rate, to correct the balance.

(c) Already many thousands of sufferers from diabetes wear pumps which can deliver a steady stream of insulin. This method keeps the amount of insulin in their blood much more constant, and it is thought that it will produce fewer long-term diabetic complications than when insulin is given by injections once or twice a day. A much smaller implantable version of the pump is being developed.

(d) At the moment one idea is that a suitable implantable reservoir might consist of a bag with a silicon rubber surface. Silicon can be punctured without producing a permanent leak, so implanted just below the skin it could be refilled, say once a month.

The power to drive the pump and operate the bio-sensor might come from a battery which could be recharged by microwaves from a coil placed above the skin.

Eyes

There is no near prospect of a transplant or artificial replacement of the whole eye. Some work using a television tube with electrodes planted into the brain has been done, but the fact that connections would need to be made in the brain for a disability that is not a threat to life make it a real problem area. However, artificial lenses are very much with us.

Cataract is a disease in which the lens of the eye gradually becomes clouded with flecks which scatter the light, rather like frosted glass. It is most common in the elderly, although it can affect even babies. It is a disease for which there is a very successful spare part. The normal lens of the eye is a lozenge of transparent jelly-like substance, held in position in a capsule with muscles which can change its shape to alter the focal length. When cataract develops in the lens it can simply be removed from its capsule and replaced by a small plastic lens which gives clear vision, although of course the muscles can no longer change the focus. The operation to remove the clouded lens of the eye has been carried out for centuries, but in the past, and still in many parts of the world, no implant is used, and the eye can only work properly with the help of thick 'pebble' glasses. The idea that pieces of plastic could be put into the eye itself only occurred to doctors when they noticed after the Second World War that perspex (Plexiglas) fragments from shattered aircraft canopies did not set up an angry reaction.

- and ears

The outer portion of the ear picks up sounds from the air and channels them towards the eardrum, which vibrates. These vibrations are amplified by a series of three tiny bones in the middle ear and then passed on to the hearing organ proper, the cochlea. This is a chamber shaped like a snail shell, and along the length of the coil is an inner membrane chamber containing an array of tiny bundles of hairs which pick up the vibrations and pass them on to the auditory nerve in the form of an electric current. Different sections of this array of hairs are disturbed by different frequencies of sound, so by working out where among the hair cells the signal to the auditory nerve comes from, the brain can tell what

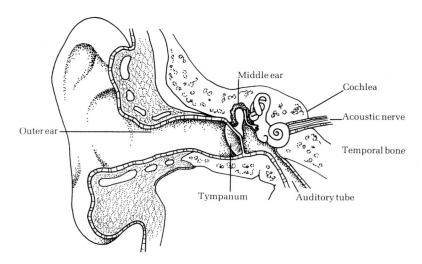

The structure of the ear. The electrodes of the artificial ear are in direct contact with the part of the acoustic nerve that is inside the cochlea

Middle ear

Cochlea

Acoustic nerve

Outer ear

Temporal bone

Tympanum

Auditory tube

frequency of sound to 'hear'. Loudness depends on the number and distribution of nerve fibres being stimulated.

There are many different causes of deafness, ranging from blocked tubes at one end to failure of the cochlea to develop at the other. Many can be treated, and replacement of one or more of the three tiny bones in the middle ear with man-made substitutes is one well-established and successful operation. If the problem is not curable, then for partial deafness a hearing aid is the usual answer. But there is no hearing aid that can treat profound, or total, deafness, which is often due to a failure of the hair cells in the cochlea. It is to help people with this problem that the 'bionic ear' has been developed. The idea is to bypass the whole of the ear and feed electric signals directly to the auditory nerve.

Sounds are picked up by a small microphone usually located some-where near the ear. They are then sent to a processor, about the size of a pack of cards, which can sit in a shirt pocket. This converts the sound signal into a pattern of electrical impulses and sends them to a transmission coil behind the ear which communicates by induction with another coil implanted immediately below the skin. From there the pattern of impulses is fed to one or more electrodes implanted in the cochlea in contact with the auditory nerve.

Many devices of this sort have been fitted in various parts of the world with varying success. Some reports have suggested that the sound signals are good enough for the individual to hold a limited telephone conversation; others say that the limit of the implant is likely to be that it helps with lip-reading. The big question now is how many separate electrodes will give the best resolution of sound. The number varies from one electrode, which will give a single input for any mix of frequencies of sound, to 24 carrying different frequences and stimulating different parts of the cochlea. Most people think that one is not enough, but that there is no great advantage in as many as 24. The optimum number may well turn out to be about six.

Although cochlear implants can be used even in the very young, many doctors who look after deaf children are doubtful. They think that the children will learn to manage better without them; and implanting a device now may mean that the cochlea is damaged, so that if better implants are developed in the next few years those children may be unable to benefit from them. For those few totally deaf children a single electrode planted on the outside surface of the cochlea gives some sensation of sound, leaving the possibility of a better implant later.

Fallopian tubes: test tube babies

In a normally fertile woman, once a month an egg comes to maturity in one of her ovaries and is released. It is gathered up by the free end of the fallopian tube and transported towards the uterus. Meanwhile a sperm may be on its way via the cervix and uterus. If they meet it is in the fallopian tube, where the sperm penetrates the egg and fertilizes it. If all

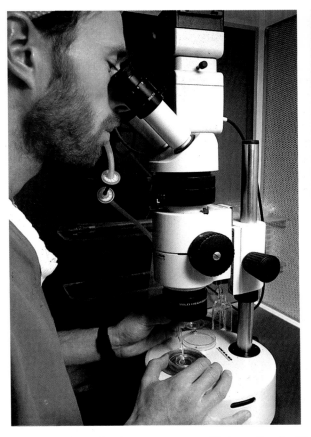

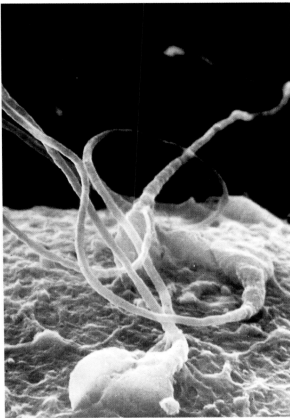

ABOVE LEFT The artificial fallopian tube. The sperm is added to the egg in the in-vitro fertilization laboratory. If the meeting is a success the resulting embryo will be returned to the mother's uterus where it may implant and grow.
ABOVE RIGHT A highly significant moment in the creation of a new life. The sperm meets the egg

goes well then the fertilized egg carries on its way to the uterus where it implants itself in the wall and begins to develop. To produce a test-tube baby, the part of the process that happens in the tube is taken over and conducted in a glass dish. The woman normally takes hormones so that when she ovulates she will produce more than one egg, which improves the odds on success. The eggs are collected as they are released from the ovary (this is done through a laparoscope) and mixed with the husband's sperm. When a sperm has penetrated an egg it is put to incubate until the genetic material of the two has united and the resulting cell has divided two or three times. After that the embryo is examined to make sure that it is developing properly, and then it is put into the uterus where it implants itself and continues its life, ultimately to be born in the normal way.

It all sounds very simple, but it only works when conditions are perfect, and a great deal of effort went into discovering the correct methods and the best time to transfer the growing foetus back into the womb.

There is still no agreement about the correct number of eggs to return to the mother to increase the chances of success without producing too many multiple births. In women who are no more than 35 years old success is expected with about 20 per cent of embryos that are actually transferred to their mothers, although not all women who attempt to have test tube babies get that far.

Organ transplants

The possibility that an organ can be successfully transplanted depends not only on the technical difficulty of the operation itself, but more on whether or not it is possible to prevent the recipient's body rejecting the new organ. It is here that the protective immune system becomes a real menace. Apart from blood, the first human tissue to be regularly transplanted was the cornea, the front surface of the eye. The cornea can be damaged when the tear system breaks down, allowing it to dry up, and when that happens the front of the eye becomes opaque, just like skin.

It is a convenient piece of tissue to transplant because it has no blood vessels to be joined up; it receives all its nutrition by diffusion from the surrounding tissues. This lack of blood vessels not only makes the cornea easy to transplant, it also means that it is not rejected by the immune system as other tissue can be, because very few lymphocytes ever get near enough to detect it. So there are no matching problems, and donated corneas can be frozen or preserved in some other way and kept in eye banks for years.

The kidney

The kidney was the first of the major organs of the body to be transplanted, and there are many reasons why this was the pioneering operation. Thousands of people suffer from total kidney failure in Britain every year, and it is incurable; the kidney can operate without nerve connections which are destroyed in any transplant operation; dialysis can maintain patients temporarily, so they can be kept alive until a really suitable kidney is available, and dialysis is also able to rescue them if the transplant fails; it is possible to minimize the rejection problems by using kidneys from closely related live donors, because we each have two kidneys and donors can manage perfectly well with one – the remaining kidney grows to accommodate the extra load; the kidney can be kept on ice for at least 24 hours without suffering irreversible damage.

The operation itself is not technically difficult, since it usually involves joining only three vessels, an artery, a vein and the ureter. The failed kidney does not even have to be removed, because the transplant is not put into the proper place but in the groin, and it is not joined into the bloodstream in the same way as a normal kidney. So the most difficult bit of the operation is removing the kidney when the donor is a live relative. The success rate of kidney transplants is now very high: 90 per cent of patients survive for one year, by which time the main danger of rejection is past. One thousand kidney transplants a year are now done in Britain, and if there were sufficient donor kidneys a further thousand lives might be saved.

Heart and lungs

The second most common organ transplant is now the heart. At first there was considerable doubt about whether a heart could manage without its nerve supply, but experiments soon showed that although a transplanted heart did react rather more slowly than a normal one, that was the least of the problems. The heart appears to be much more vulnerable to rejection than the kidney, and if it fails it can do so suddenly with no possibility of rescue, so a much closer watch has to be kept for rejection. This means taking regular samples of tissue from the heart after the operation, and repeated bouts of rejection, even if they are corrected, can damage the blood vessels and result in a fatal build-up of fatty deposits inside the arteries. Because of these and other problems most of the early heart transplant patients died, but ways have been found of controlling this and now in some centres seven out of ten patients survive for over a year.

The heart and lungs often go wrong together, since they are very closely linked. If the heart is not pumping properly then the lungs may become congested and irreparably damaged. Sometimes blood vessels in the lungs become narrowed or congested first, and then the right side of the heart may fail because it is having to pump too hard to push the blood into the lungs. For people with these problems there would be no point in transplanting only the heart or the lungs – the only solution is both. Heart–lung transplants suffer from all the same difficulties as transplants of the heart alone, only more so. When the lungs are re-moved they have to be kept partially inflated as well as cooled. The length of time they can be kept safely outside the body is thought to be measured in minutes rather than hours; and rejection is even more of a problem than with hearts. There is also a special difficulty that is peculiar to the lungs. For some reason lungs that have been deprived of blood, even for a few minutes, later suffer a strange stiffening, which may happen some time after the operation, after the lungs have been working well for days. Fortunately if the patient is put on to a respirator for a while the stiffness wears off.

The liver

Transplanting the liver is technically much more difficult than the kidney or heart. It is a large organ, extremely active biochemically, and the transplant operation is an anaesthetist's nightmare. Just one of the problems is that, like other organs, the liver is kept on ice between removal and transplanting. As it is put into its new body and begins to work its cells leak large quantities of potassium, and a rise in potassium can stop the heart. So the anaesthetist has to correct it. No sooner has he done so than the recovering liver cells begin to take the potassium back in again, so once again the salt balance is upset. Liver transplant pa-tients always lose a great deal of blood – one centre will only operate with 17 litres (30 pt) of blood standing by – and the large quantity of foreign blood, which has been treated to prevent clotting, causes extra trouble for the kidneys and heart. This means that the surgeon some-

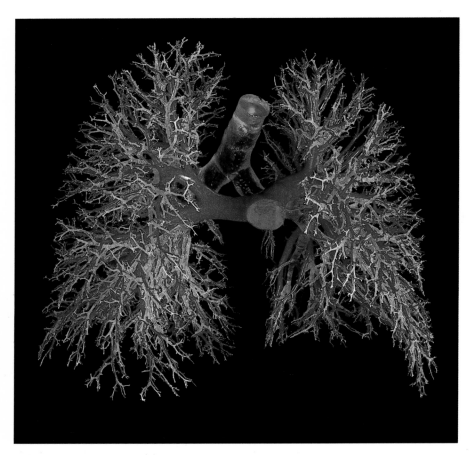

The blood vessels of the heart and lungs. Casts like these are formed by filling the vessels with resin

times has to put the patient on a heart–lung machine. And he has other problems. Not only does he have more vessels to join up, some of them difficult to get at, but one of the vessels is the bile duct. In the wrong place bile is a most unpleasant substance which has a tendency to digest any exposed tissue, so the join in the duct is likely to be digested. Some of the earliest liver transplant patients died as a result of this, but surgeons have now found a way of protecting the join in the duct with a temporary lining until it has healed well enough to defend itself from its corrosive contents. The only advantage the liver transplant team have is that for some reason the body seems less inclined to reject a foreign liver than many other organs.

The pancreas and the islets of Langerhans
Pancreas transplants are still really at the experimental stage. Unlike the liver they are proving to be exceptionally vulnerable to rejection; the great majority fail within a year. One reason for attempting a pancreas transplant is to treat diabetes which, as we have seen, is caused by the failure of the pancreas to produce insulin. Not all of the pancreas is

involved in insulin production, only clumps of specialized cells called the islets of Langerhans, which are scattered throughout the organ. One obvious step is to transplant only the islets, but unfortunately they, too, are very likely to be rejected. However, it now appears that the antigen that causes rejection may not be on the cells of the islets themselves, but on lymph cells which have been included with the islets in the transplanted tissue, so the next step is to kill these cells with antibodies before transplanting the islet cells.

The brain

The idea of transplanting a brain is a thoroughly uncomfortable one; apart from any other considerations, who would be the donor and who the recipient? Fortunately it is as unlikely as it is unattractive. But even if there is no prospect of anybody ever installing a transplanted brain and remaking all its nerve connections, the idea of transplanting brain cells is not at all absurd; it has already been done in rats, and a step towards it has been taken in humans.

One in a hundred people over 60 suffer from Parkinsonism, a disease in which they gradually lose control of their movements. A sufferer's hands can become so shaky that he cannot even pick up a glass of water. The reason for this loss of control is inside the brain itself. There are chemicals called neurotransmitters which allow messages to be sent from one part of the nervous system to another. One of these chemicals, called dopamine, is a vital part of the system that allows the brain to direct movement. It is made by a particular group of cells at the base of the brain, and in people with Parkinson's disease for some reason these cells have died. The purpose of the brain tissue transplant would be to implant enough living cells of the type that make dopamine to restore the communication to normal. Most experiments so far have been done in rats, transplanting brain cells from rat foetuses. Foetal cells are used because they are expected to grow links into the brain better than adult cells would, and are less likely to be rejected. Many of these experimental grafts have taken well, and not only a form of rat Parkinsonism but also other types of brain damage in rats have been corrected. In the human experiments the dopamine-produced cells did not come from a foetus. There are other cells in the body that produce dopamine. They are in the adrenal gland just above the kidney, and the human patients had transplants of cells taken from their own adrenals. The results of these human tests were disappointing, so this is a long way from becoming the standard treatment. However, in case it does prove valuable, and it is found that it is necessary to use foetal cells, rather than those from the adrenals, researchers are already trying to find ways of growing the cells in tissue culture in the laboratory. Otherwise, even if using foetal tissue for such a purpose were regarded as ethical, it would never be possible to find anything like enough cells for all those who might need them.

Preventing rejection

One advantage brain cell transplants have over others is that the brain appears to be a safe area as far as the immune system is concerned, so the rejection of the transplant is impossible, or at least much less likely. But apart from the cornea all other transplants call for a delicate balancing act, between the dangers of rejection and the risk of making the immune system so helpless that the patient dies of infectious disease or cancer, or one of the other side effects of immuno-suppressive drugs. It is mainly advances in handling rejection that have improved the success rate of all transplants.

Tissue typing

The first step in preventing rejection is tissue typing. This means checking that the selection of HLA antigens carried by the cells of the donor and recipient are as similar as possible (see page 000). The fewer different antigens they have, the less chance there is that the immune system will react with a massed attack on the intruder. HLA antigens are part of the genetic inheritance, and close relatives are therefore likely to have very similar tissue types; that is one reason why the success of kidney transplants between close relatives has always been so much better than the others.

To check the tissue type, the immunologists mix the person's cells with antibodies to as many as they can of the range of possible antigens, together with some complement which will attack the cell if once it is labelled by the antibody. The test is done on a plate with masses of tiny wells with a different antibody in each. Then the plates are checked for dead cells, because any cells that have been killed must be carrying the antigen matching the antibody in that well. The test is done on the blood of both donor and recipient, and then the results are compared. They will not be identical, even between close relatives, except in the case of identical twins. So even with a reasonably good match the immune system of the person receiving the transplant has to be considerably suppressed.

Immunosuppression

To reject a transplanted organ the immune cells have to be able to divide and produce large numbers of copies of themselves; so to stop that happening drugs are used that will interfere with dividing cells. Many of these drugs were actually developed to treat cancer, where once again the need is for a substance that is lethal to fast-growing cells. Often they have serious side effects, apart from making the body much more vulnerable to infection, so it is difficult to find the right balance between the opposing dangers of rejection or damage to other organs. One discovery that has made a great deal of difference, particularly in heart and heart-lung transplants, is the drug Cyclosporin-A. It comes from a strain of fungus, and was first studied as a possible antibiotic. It was not a particularly useful antibiotic, but it turned out later that it did interfere powerfully with the immune reaction. It appears to be much more selective in its action than other immuno-suppressives, attacking only the T- and B-lymphocytes that have just been switched on, ready to begin multiplying and go into action against the new transplant. It is still not the perfect answer, because it can be harmful to the kidneys, and there may be an even better way.

The most selective method of preventing organ rejection is still experimental; it uses the immune system itself. As soon as signs of rejection appear following a transplant, the doctors take from a sample of the patient's blood some of the active white cells which are involved in rejection of the transplanted organ. They grow antibodies to these in the cells of mice, then inject these mouse antibodies into the patient's bloodstream where they should hunt out and disable the cells involved in the rejection.

WHERE NEXT?

Until very recently scientific medicine developed in an atmosphere of universal approval, and the doctor and his colleague the scientist were the modern 'knights in shining armour'. Their achievements have been remarkable: because of vaccination and antibiotics we no longer fear infectious disease; because of improved understanding, deficiency diseases like diabetes and anaemia can be appropriately treated; because of improved techniques and anaesthetics, surgery of all kinds is much safer; treatment of some cancers, particularly those which attack children and young people, is increasingly successful. By any standards the record is impressive.

But during the 1970s and '80s doubts have been expressed about how far medicine can go in this direction. One problem is cost, because much of modern treatment is very expensive. Criticism has concentrated on money spent on heroic surgery like heart transplants, yet some medical treatments with expensive courses of drugs can cost even more. Because of the way medical treatment is funded in the National Health Service, problems associated with the cost of 'high-tech' medicine have come into focus in Britain earlier than in many other countries. Nevertheless it is rapidly becoming clear that there is virtually no limit to the amount of a country's wealth that health care could eat up, and the more medicine can do, the more resources it is capable of absorbing.

Partly because of this cost there are criticisms that medicine concentrates too exclusively on *curing* disease; much more effort should be put into prevention. However, the two great 'epidemics' of our time, cancer and heart disease, are proving very difficult for the medical profession to prevent. There is no 'vaccination' against cancer or heart disease, and preventive steps that might be taken are more for individuals (giving up smoking and changing diet), or governments (improving the environment and changing price structures which at present favour unhealthy foods). Nevertheless a great deal of work is now going into research aimed at establishing the causes of the diseases and identifying the individuals who are most at risk.

But scientific medicine has also found itself under attack for another, more unexpected reason. Doctors are accused of concentrating too hard on measurement and machines and ignoring the 'whole patient'. This has led some individuals to reject the advice of orthodox doctors and turn towards some form of alternative medicine. The record of achievement of scientific medicine makes it clear that there is no sense in the suggestion that medicine should move away from the strict evaluation of the results of any new treatment; and where there have been comparative tests of the efficacy of the two approaches, like the trial of the homeopathic cure, rhus tox, against mainstream anti-inflammatory drugs, the mainstream drug won conclusively. Nevertheless many doctors accept that there is a lesson to be learned from this swing against them; that they have been in danger of forgetting how the attitude and state of mind of an individual patient can affect the success of even the most scientific of treatment.

ILLUSTRATION SOURCES

Professor D.J. Allison, Department of Diagnostic Radiology, Royal Postgraduate Medical School, Hammersmith, London: 90-91, 93 (above) (3), 93 (below)
Amersham International plc: 96 (right)
Heather Angel: 66
Sue Baker: 9, 21 (right), 32, 38 (left), 44, 51 (taken from Ronald Melzack and Patrick D. Wall The Challenge of Pain, revised ed. 1982. Reprinted by permission of Penguin Books Ltd), 54 (below), 107 (below), 109 (left), 117 (below)
BBC Hulton Picture Library: 13 (left), 27 (above)
Biophoto Associates, Leeds: 79 (2), 112
BPCC/Aldus Books: 90 (left)
Paul Brierley: 59 (right)
British Museum, London: 26
Dr S. Bown, University College Hospital, London: 6 (below)
Camera Press Ltd: 36 (Walter Castro), 60 (right)
J.-L. Carmet, Paris: 55 (below)
Professor L. Caro: 62 (left) (first published Journal of Bacteriology, 100: 1091-1104, 1985)
Chester Beatty Research Institute: 47
Bruce Coleman Ltd: 54 (above) (Eric Crichton)
Colorific!: 111 (left) (Black Star), 115 (left) (John Moss)
Dr P.B. Cotton, Middlesex Hospital, London: 85 (2)
Cromwell Hospital IVF LAB, London: 119 (left)
Department of Medical Photography, Institute of Urology, London: 6 (above), 84
Department of Medical Photography, St Bartholomew's Hospital, London: 96 (left)
Department of Radiology, University College Hospital, London: 20

Martin Dohrn: Frontispiece, Title Page, 8, 20, 38 (right), 55 (above), 74, 90-1, 93 (above) (3), 93 (below), 94, 98, 105, 111 (right), 115 (right), 119 (left), 122
Mary Evans Picture Library: 49
Infinity Features, Hank Morgan: 109 (right)
Institute of Obstetrics and Gynaecology, Hammersmith Hospital, London: 83
C. James Webb: 59 (left)
London Lithotripter Centre: 86 (2)
Ludwig Institute for Cancer Research, Cambridge: 42
The Mansell Collection, London: 30
McDonnell Douglas (photo courtesy of NASA): 71
The Middlesex Hospital, London: 21 (left)
MRC Hammersmith Hospital, London: 18 (right)
MRI Unit, Hammersmith Hospital, London: 23 (below) (2)
National Hospital for Nervous Diseases, London: 14, 17, 74
National Institute for Medical Research, The Ridgeway, Mill Hill, London NW7 1AA (scanning electron micrograph by K. Sullivan, P.M. Taylor and B.A. Askonas): 35
Oxford Magnet Technology Ltd: 23 (above)
Philips Medical Systems: 99
Popperfoto: 60 (left)
Rand Rocket: 115 (right)
Barry Richards: 13 (right)
Ann Ronan Picture Library, London: 50, 95
The Royal College of Surgeons: Title Page, 122
Royal Free Hospital, Mr J.D. Abrams: 81
Royal Marsden Hospital, Sutton: 94, 98
Royal National Orthopaedic Hospital, Stanmore,

INDEX

Numbers in *italics* refer to illustrations